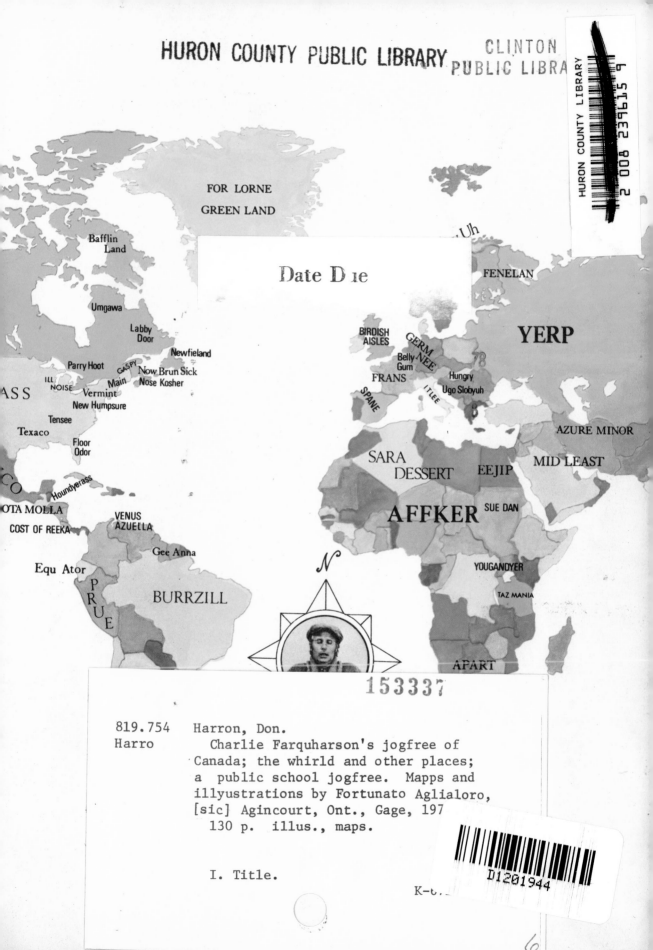

FOR LORNE GREEN LAND

Bafflin Land

Umgawa

Labby Door

Newfieland

Parry Hoot
GASPY
Now Brun Sick
ILL NOISE
Main
Nose Kosher
Vermint
New Humpsure

Tensee

Texaco

Floor Odor

ASS

CO

OTA MOLLA

COST OF REEKA

Houndyerass

VENUS AZUELLA

Gee Anna

Equ Ator

P R U E

BURRZILL

Date D ie

Uh

FENELAN

YERP

BIRDISH AISLES

GERM NEE
Belly Gum
FRANS
78
Hungry
Ugo Slobyuh
ITLEE
SPANE

AZURE MINOR

SARA DESSERT

EEJIP

MID LEAST

AFFKER

SUE DAN

YOUGANDYER

TAZ MANIA

APART

N

153337

819.754
Harro

Harron, Don.
Charlie Farquharson's jogfree of
Canada; the whirld and other places;
a public school jogfree. Mapps and
illyustrations by Fortunato Aglialoro,
[sic] Agincourt, Ont., Gage, 197
130 p. illus., maps.

I. Title.

K-o.

6

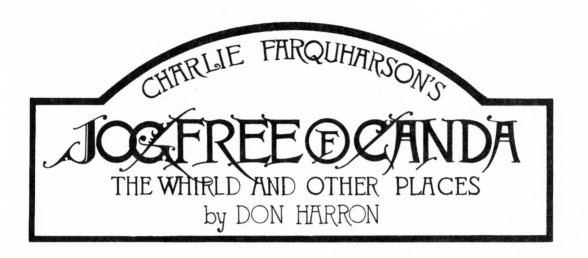

CHARLIE FARQUHARSON'S
JOGFREE ℹ CANDA
THE WHIRLD AND OTHER PLACES
by DON HARRON

A Pubic School Jogfree

———

Autherized by yer Depart
Mentals of Edification
Fur Use in Pubic, High,
And Continyation Schools

———

Mapps and Illyustrations by Fortunato Aglialoro (con gusto)

GAGE PUBLISHING

Enturd accordion to yer Act of Parlmint
in th'Office of yer Minster of Aggerculture
by Charles Ewart Farquharson, D.O.P.E. *

*Docter of Personnel Expeerients
(Honerdairy Degree, Trench U.   '73)

er yer Toyola Coronary. He figgers he'd breed them in the fall, raze them all winter and spring, and in the summer he'd train these big fellas to lie still in the waters of the Bay. Then he'd sell them to the Amurkens as off-shore Ilands.

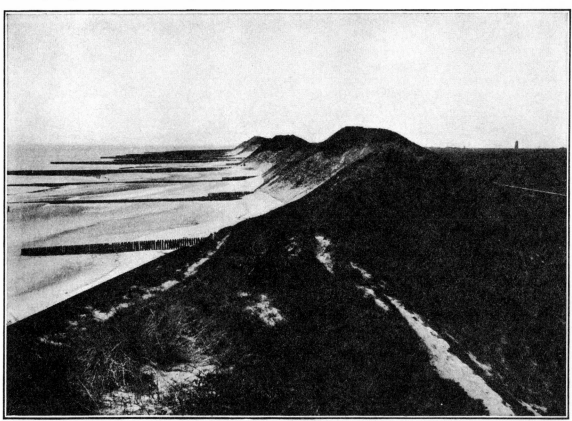

Dykes on the beech

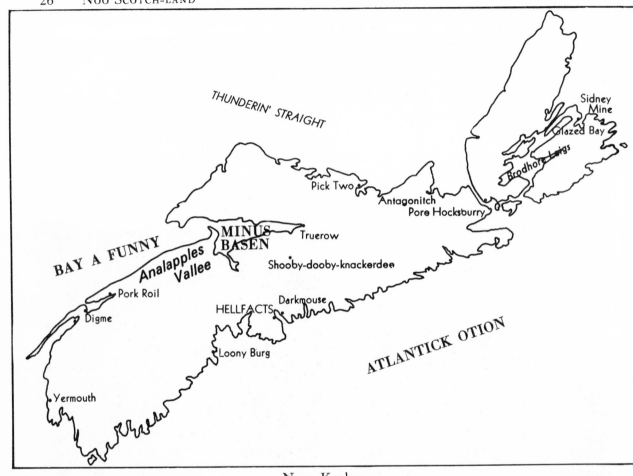

Nose Kosher

NOSE KOSHER

Nose Kosher is what yer old-time Latins say when they mean yer Noo Scotch-land. Mind you, the reel Noo Scotch is over in Newfieland and called Screech, on accounta that's what ya do when ya gits a mouthfull.

Yer Scotch cum over here becuz they was so indetted to yer Anglish. They settle down when they seen Nose Kosher's deeply indentured coastline, fer they was used to bein' inner-ears back home.

Seems yer Nose Kosherer farmer jist can't win. It's too wet fur weet, so the only thing to do is feeld yer oats. Barley makes a livin'. Fer yeers they bin tryna git the salt water outa the land with furtlizer. But now it's the vicey of yer versey. With them City Oil Slickers sinking ther shafts all around yer Stable Island, yer Marntider farmer is now worried about all that crap

gittin' into the sea. I think the only way out is fer to sudsidy-ize the poor fella with what they call yer Garnteed Anual Increment, fer to offset all the other stuff he has to put up with . . . yer Garnteed Anual Excrement.

You take yer avrage farm, Hants County in yer Rotten Hills. Yer soiled samples is so pore 'bout all a man kin cultyvate is his frends, until he gits plowed under by taxes. Mind you, there's a few paltry fellas turn out to be not too bad with the chicks. Aigs is sold down to yer Boston States, force-fed into yer Kernel Sandy chicken, and sole back to yer Martimes at much hire prizes. This makes yer farmer down there wonder if he's his brooder's keeper.

But most Nose Koshers feel that they're ther kipper's brother, and they lern to trawl even before they kin walk. But that don't work out too good neether, fer most dipsy fishermen spend mosta ther time cleenin' the fish, wile the hole-sailers on land do the same thing to them. Yer cleened fish is layed on yer dry-doc till it becum Fish Flakes, a poplar Martime breckfist food.

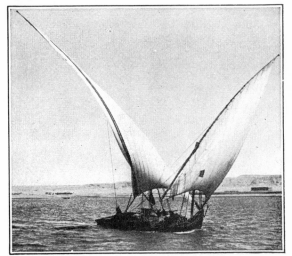

Yer Bloonose Flying Nun

Martimers is prowd of ther fission boats. Most of all yer BLEWNOSE, wich used to be in its Cups all over the whirled and wich was took over by a Broor who tuk it outa the foam and put it O'land. It has since bin tuk back by yer Reganal Guvmint, where it remanes today as yer Gratest Dory Ever Sold.

Nose Kosher is pritty, and I gess Peggy's Coze has the prittiest part. That's wher all yer water-cullered artists go down to do her in oil . . . wich is what Premeer Riggin clames Pee-Air Turdo is tryna do to him, with his big rig.

Down yer coast is yer Germn settlement of Looneybuggers, wich cum over a couple centurions ago, but sum seem to be still "stricken yer doych." Even them as speaks broken Canadyun seems to tack on a U at the end of what they say . . . like "when you wanna mate wit my ram, U?", or "Yer boy gonna go up Mount Allison, U?"*

*UPPER FEETNOTE: Altho' if they was goin' in fer yer hire edification, they'd more'n likely hed fer yer Dollhousey U.

Up Cake Briton way is yer Minors, and they work harder'n Hellfacts. Yer Cake Britner is ruff and ruggered, jist like yer Cabbitch Trale, and he has to go undyground fer to make a good minor livin', altho' some does it by strippin'. Round yer Brodhore Laigs you kin hear the lokal inhibitants speek with the Garlic (yer old High scotch tung). And they even dun it over the raddio till that CBC Resident-in-charge-of-yer-Vice, Listless Stinkler, cut ther wire off.

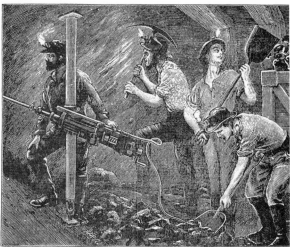

Minors with coalmen lamps

Mosta yer cole mines is under yer salty waters, and they hafta take out four ton a a water fur every ton a cole, wich is why they thot they shud git outa yer cole-bizness and into yer hevvyer water. So the Guvmint give some Amerken signtist four millyun dollers for his resspee. So far they've made water, but she ain't hevvy enuff to sell. It gits hevvy in the winter when she freezes, but that don't cut no ice down in yer States.

I think that's wher yer Leader of yer Opposite Position, Bob Stansfeeld, got the idee fer his last 'lection campain. He figgered if he froze our wages off fer ninety days in yer erly fall, why he cud sell that much more undyware.

But it's cole and steal that still makes the munny in yer Sidny's Mind, not yer Nukuler Fishin'. They say that if all yer

Caked Briton cole fer one yeer was loded on one trane, she'd be more'n a thousand mile long. (And more'n likely shunted onto a side-in wile the guvmint tries to make up it's mind about makin' more water till they finely start yer Hevvy trip.)

Many yer Martimers makes minin' his bizness. Up yer Analapples Vallee they got a Gypsum* mine makin' seement, stucko, plasterd, and wall-bored (used hed-on by peeple what drink wall-bangers).

Pugwatch, hard by yer Antagonitch, has got Salt Mines owned by yer Serious Eatin, the Commonist millyunair.** He uses his own salt fer to put the blocks to his cattle, fer he's over eighty and still showin' his calfs all over yer whirled. He sez yer salt is also good fer curing hay, but of what he don't tell.

There's lots more to Nose Kosher. Yer cotton ballers at Yarnmuth. Yer Music Festeral at Shooby-dooby-knackerdee. Yer navel scenter at Darkmouse,*** jist acrost yer Anguish All Macdonalds Britch from Hellfacts.

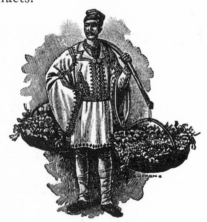

Yer Analapples Vallee fruit

You shud see Hellfacts, known to yer servicemen during Whirled War Eleven by the name of Atholevill.**** It's got the oldest things in Canda you'll ever see, speshully that over the hill Sitty-del, wich is an old fartficiation now used in yer dry season by Helluvagonians as a nice place fer to git grass stanes on ther neeze. You'll find it's a hill where yer locals is inklined to do anything s'long as it's not on the level.

****WORETIME FEETNOTE: When strangers called it that, yer avrage Helluvagonian wud ask: "Jist passin' thru?"

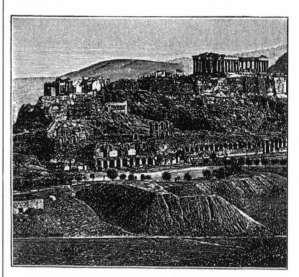

Sittydell Hill

(curtsy Nose Kosher Chambre of Commers)

*CROSST FEETNOTE: The workers call it yer "Sum Gyp" mine.

**LEFT FEETNOTE: Now he's not one of them Eatin's has the big store in Trawntuh. That'd be yer first and second Timothy Eatin's bilt that church in Holy Timothy Square to St. Timothy and all Eatin's to yer grater glory of Tim Eatin in loving memry of God.

***WET FEETNOTE: Called yer *H.M.S. Sheerwater*, but most Darkmice peefur to take it strait.

For Trish

TABLE OF CONTENTS

JIST ANOTHER PREE-FACE

I rite books when it's too wet to plow. This spring we had forty days of precipituss-pie-tation and sixty days of electionrearing, and between the two I put my nose into this book. Ornerily I'm a mixed farmer, dirt and derry . . . I never made much of a livin off of eether, but my favrit subjeck, Jogfree, is mostly dirt . . . and that seams to be what sells today . . . you take that book by that girl from the Marsh, yer X-rated Riviera Hollander, she rit all about how to git weeds outa yer garden, "The Happy Ho-er." But I figger with my sense of humus, I could give you the reel dirt. So here is "Charlie Farquharson's Jogfree Book," some soiled matter decomposed all by myself. Jist like spreadin' time, I think it purty well covers the ground.

C.E.F.*

R.R. #2,
Between the Lines (9th and 10th)
On yer Fift Sideroad
Metropopolitan Parry Sound

INNERDUCKSHUN

This book is not on yer curlicyoulum of yer Alimentary schools fer to help the boys and girls matrickle-late together. Jogfree is not tot any more, having bin nash-nalized along with Histry into a Combine called yer Socialist Studdys.** (Follow these Assricks down blow to yer Feetsnote.) But Histry is not Jogfree, nor the vice of yer versey. Jogfree is what we had to start with, and Histry is the genral mess we made of it. I think it's time to take stock agin and see if we can't do better with anuther run at yer second wind.

I don't want to be a teecher's pest, but if there's anything you don't understand, I xplaned it at the back of my A-pendix. But being Gaged to a cheep publisher, they cut the thing out.

Anyways, Jogfree has never bin a lavveratory subjeck, but needs several feel trips on the side (wich I always finds works out better than trying to make it back to the house).

I wood like to desecrate this book to my boy Orville, who never herd of Jogfree and thot it was jist runnin' around loose, wich he has bin doin' reglar weekends since he turned sexteen. I hope he looks at the maps and grafts anyways, fer, as they say in yer Adversetise-ments, a pitcher is worth a thousand blerbs.

---

*Charles Ewart Farquharson and not yer Canadyan Exhibitionery Force, altho he was part of that, too, as Private Second class in yer Royal Muskoka Dismounted Foot, in Whirled War Eleven.

**DUBBLEBED FEETSNOTE: I spose that'd be yer Daisy Lewis tellin Pee-air Turdo what to do all that time they was shackled up together in yer Common House.

Part One: Yer Hole

CHAP ONE: JOGFREE: YER ALIMENTAREES

Jogfree is a look at how yer Erth's form is filled out by the natural bounders of its continence. We wull spend some time on the water circumsizing us, but mostly fer to git at yer climaxtick effeck.

Jogfree don't have too much to do with yuman beans, wich I s'pose puts it purty much in a class by itself. Mind you, there wudn't be no Jogfree without some yuman bean fer to studdy it, jist as yer mountin ain't reely one till it's bin mounted by eether man er goat. And goats don't git much outa Jogfree less you throw the book at them and then they die-jest it in ther own way.

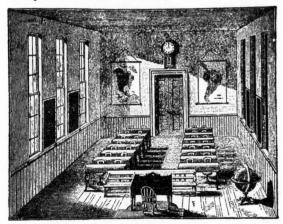

In a class by itself

CHAP TWO: YER ERTH IN YER SOLER SISTERN

Most peeple think the whirled is a ball, but they'd be mostly yer teeny agers. After they git old, they'll find out it's a bit flat at both ends. That's on accounta finely gittin' dizzy resolving on its own axes. Some Jograffers call the hole Erth with yer flat Poles a Oblate's Fearoid, but that sounds to me like Cathlick Poppygander.

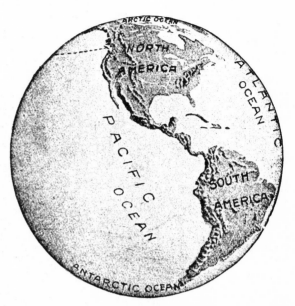

Yer Westend Hemisfearyoid

I hate to tell you this, but yer Erth is not the senter of yer Soler Sistern. It's jist a small dark objeck spaced out among yer other plants, like Murkry, Marse, and Venis. None of them is too lifely ether, on accounta we is all fixed stars, cut off before our primetime by the great Vetnary-Aryan-in-the-sky giving us the final spade.

CHAP THREE: YER SON

These plants is jist sons of yer Son, havin' bin thrown off from yer Soler's Plexus during a gas attack. The fack that yer Erth is manely made up of hard, cold gas makes you wunder wear yer shortage come from. A Son, by deafnishun, is a large mass of hot gas that shines by its own light. (I got one, too, name of Orville.)

Like it er not, yer Son is not the big cheese neether.* We used to think it was the biggest star in our blue hevven, on

*GREEN FEETSNOTE: Some peeple think the moon still is.

accounta it's the sentral heeting fer the rest of us. But it jist happens to be only the hottest thing in our Gal-Ex-Laxy.*

The rest of us plants is just dead bodies hoovering around yer Son's oar-bit, and by hinkus yer Son must be one boiler room of a place. Sides bein' a millyun times bigger'n Erth, it's more'n a thousand times in heat. The figgers is Assternomic (wich means far out), but on the face of it I'd say was ten thousand Fornheat . . . give er take a deegree.

See thru a glass darkly during yer E-clips and you'll find yer Son has a lot more goin' fer it than peers on the surfs. What looks like yer overdun frydegg is reely yer Son's Corona Corona, wich sounds to me like a lotta blue smoke but is realy a millyun miles of gas on fire. And that's what gits lit up yer Northend lights, also known as yer Boring Alice at Aurora.

F & P Astronomical, Calgary, Alta.

Yer overdun Son

CHAP FOUR: YER PLANTS

As I sed before, yer plants begun as jist spots offa yer Son and grew cold till they become big Cosmical blackheds. And the more far out in yer Universal they flu, the bigger they got fer their boots. Let's start with yer nearest to yer Son and most compact, Murkry.

*HOT FEETSNOTE: Yer Galexlaxy is a tecknickle term fer our pertickler bar of yer Milky Way.

Murkry: Most peeple don't think of Murkry as yer avrage Compact, but she's yer smallest and most hothouse of yer plants. On accounta the heat's on all the time, there's some as says the place has no atmosfear. That seems kinda mean to say when nobuddy has ever give it a visit. There's no tellin' what some wimmen asternuts could do with a little ulteerier deck-ratin'.

Venis: Not so torrid and not so much in heat as you'd think. She's our nextdoor naybor and, since she's the brightest lite in our local firmaminit, she's called yer Evening Star and can be seen in the erly edition even before yer Twilit Zone.

Yer Serviet Roosians sent one of them Unmanly Spooknuts up to look at her, but nothin' could be seen on accounta yer Smog. Three of them Spaced Men got sent to Sighbeerier for this, on accounta yer Krumlin Commizars thot they'd all gone fer a dirty weekend to Loss Angles, Callfornya.

By the way, don't pay no tension to other Jogfree books. There are no canals on Venis. That'd be yer Marse.

Marse: Our naybor on t'other side. Not so much in heat, but seems to be in season as yer vegetatin seems to change from blew-green to cow-brown, wich proves that the place is more than jist desserts. It may be that yer canals is meerly melting Marse bars, but it still looks like our Trench river sisterm when seen on yer Telepathyscope.

Joopter: If youse wanta git into Steller Reelstate, buy Joopter, the biggest of yer plants. All you can catch lookin' thru yer tellyscope is a buncha Big Bands, but I hear that's all comin' back . . . yer Big Band Eara.

Slattern: Not so big as yer Joopter, but more fur out, and can row-tate rings around the rest of them. Close-up, looks like a big Frizzbee what got preggerunt.

Yeranus: Hung well back at the end of yer Universal. Seems to mind its own pees and kews and keeps its mean distants from the rest of us.

Napchewin: Sounds wet, don't it? Mebbe it gits some run-off from yer Milky Way, but it's so darn far-out nobuddy's herd from it.

Plutoe: Yer dog star, wich is mebbe why it's the furthest out-side. It may have bin a throw-off unleashed from yer Napchewin. Scientificks are not even sure if it's a plant but, bein' Plutoe, it sure leans t'word other plants.

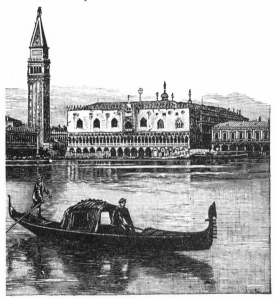

Canals on Marse

Three Fases at Eve: Yer Moon

Now let's git this strait. I don't know how to brake it to you, but every plant's gotta moon (and sometimes three er four er more) in Utter Spaceland. When you see yer Moon out the car winder, that's ars all right. But if you was studdying up yer Pastronomy in one of yer Observeyer-torys, you'd see yer plant Slattern has got ten moons. I mean all at once, not jist like ours havin' a peeriod every 29 days. Imagine what ten moons wud do to yer berth rate with all the yung cupples park-ed down by Prospeck Point watching the submarine races! Things must be jumpin' on Joopter cuz they got twelve moons, and evry one of them resolvin' to go the wrong way, jist like them kids parked down by Prospeck Point.

Nothin' much to say about our moon, sept that it travels in a illipstickle ore-bit round us and is compleatly uninhibited . . . altho' them Asternuts from yer Emission Controls did talk about comin' across a lot of differnt craters when they was gittin' the rocks off with their Loonier Model.

Other Plantoids: Cumits and Meatiers

If yuh see a long, long tale a-winding between yer heavenly dead bodies some nite, that'd be yer Cumit. They don't come too offen. We've had yer Bill Haley's purty reglar round the clock, and last year we had one that dint never show, yer Ko-hoteks. Yer Cumit is a dirty ice cube that don't hang around too long on accounta them hot gases burnin' off its tale end. But, fer a one-nite stand, you can't beat it.

Yer Meatier is smaller than yer Cumit, sort of a haff-Assteroid that probly broke off from sum other plant. My theery is that, bean so compack, yer avrage Meatier is probly a chip offa yer old Murkry.

We once had a Meatier land on the back fallow, back in 1934, and we made a little munny chargin' toureeists 25 sense a head fer to look at it. But the guvermint

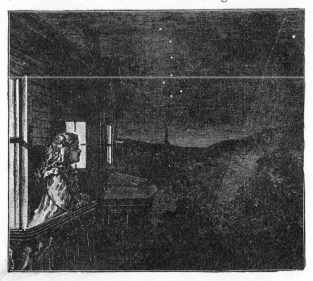

Little Nipper lookin' at Big Dipper

step in and said we hadda pay tax on the incum from our Murkry Meatier on accounta it cum from a broad and was considered Imported Iron.

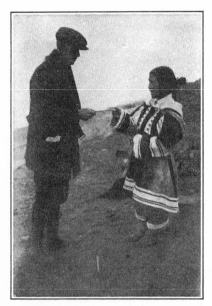

Charlie Farquharson and the Little Woman

Other flashers in yer cosmickal pan

Yer Shooty star is not a Cumit, but more of a Go-it. Jist a flash in the pan of yer Big Dippy, gitting burnt off too fast and taleing off into nothing, unlike some of our big shooty stars on Erth, like John Wane er Frank Shooter.

Yer Pole Star (And I don't mean that NH Heller, Peat Stemkowski) is the thing that's allus bein' pointed at by yer Big Diaper. It's so durn far away, the light from this North Star takes more'n forty years to git here. (I don't mean the Parry Sound *North Star*. Its news is never more than too weak old.)

Yer Queerzars is big Red fellas winking at us every millenema. We only recent got cosmick wind of them and don't know how long they bin radio active. You'd have to travel thru yer light yeers and yer dark fer to git at them, fer they're even beyond our Universal-internashunal.

Yer Flying Sorcerer is man-maid, what they call yer Unindemnifiable Flying Objeck. When Premeer Turdo whispers under his breth in the Common House at yer Leader of yer Opposite Posishun, he sez "U.F.O." This brung a lotta trubble to us United Farmers of Ontario when we had our Animal Husbandry Convention in Ottawa . . . they wunt let us put U.F.O. after our names becuze they sed it was the kinda langwidge only fit fer a Prime Minister.

CHAP FIVE: YER ASSTEROLOGY

Jogfree is s'posed to be yer studdy of yer Erth having relations with animals and peeple. But before we git back down there, we better deel with Assterolgers, who are well hung up on yer other plants, and how they put peeple under the inflooence.

Yer Assterology is writ in the papers every day and tells peeple how they can't do a thing less they check in the sodiac the constipation they was born under. But all of them horrerscopes hangs on us bein' the dead senter of yer Universal, what they call yer foke-all point. But Gala Layou, a Middle Age Eyetalian and mebbe yer erliest Optimist, invent the Biknackerlers. And sittin' up there in his Tower of Pizza, he prooved we was center-frugging around yer Son.

You'd think yer Church peeple would be glad to find out yer Son's in his Hevven, makin' it all right with the Whirled, and they could fergit about yer Horrerscopers and git back to Bingo. But nossir. Them Popes and Carnals wanted the erth to be head-and-hindquarters of yer Universal— and that's flat. And flat was the way they wanted yer Erth, too, flatter'n you-no-what on a platter. So when that Gal Alayou told them we wasn't squares no more but rounders, they disbeleeved him, even when they seen by yer loony Ee-clips that yer Erth's shadder was a sercular. They din't even bleeve it when that Porchgeese navelgator Madge-Ellen saled round yer Glow-ball and come back where he

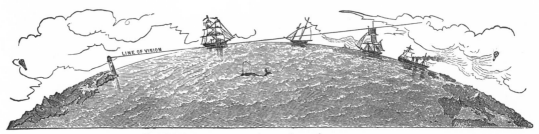

Lookin' acrost yer circuminterference

started frum. And it were done in the next Sentennial (altho' arsy-versy in a aunty-cockwisederection) by Captain Hook.

Them Assterologers are still playin' Blind Man's Bluffin' even today, when they figger we is all under the dumnation of Toreass yer Bull or Cancel yer Crabs.

CHAP SIX: YER ERTH AS A HOLE

Now that we reelize our Erth is jist one of billyuns of basketballs bouncing around in yer permamint firmamint, let's get down to it, fer it's all we got. And Yer Big Rafferee is not gonna give us a new one to start another game. It's a darn good thing Jogfree brings us down to Erth, fer it's likely the only place we can afford to go after all the moneys they spent at yer Cape Carniveral and yer Houston Assterodome.

As I said before, yer Erth looks to be a solid ball. But, like the rest of us, it's gittin' flatter on top and bigger round yer middle, ending up as a slitely de-pressed Sfear, with at leese two Hemi-sfeeroids.

I like yer Jogfree better than yer Assterology and Passtronomy because its bases is not theeries but facks. Yer facks come in two kinds: yer permamint and yer changebull. Yer reason fer studdying the permamints of Jogfree is so's you can understand why other peeple live the way they do, even tho' you yerself wunt be cot dead doin' it. The reason fer yer changebull facks is mostly Man. Fer example, yer copulation explosion. The popillation of yer avrage big sitty is

changed all the time reglar as a baby. But in yer smaller senters yer popillation figgers stays even, because in a small place every time some young girl has a baby some young fella leaves town.

Mind you, Man don't cut that much musterd in yer Jogfree. If you took all the peeples on Erth, three or four billyun, you could stick 'em in a box three quarts of a mile on all sides. And if she was hung over yer Nagger Falls and was give a push, there'd be one ring-tailed snorter of a splash fer a few secs. But after that yer Erth wood go on running, probly better'n before.

Mind you, things miten't be as lifely as when we was around kicking up yer dust, but they woodn't be quite so dethly, too. It'd jist go back to yer Survival of yer Fattest accordin' to yer Theery of yer

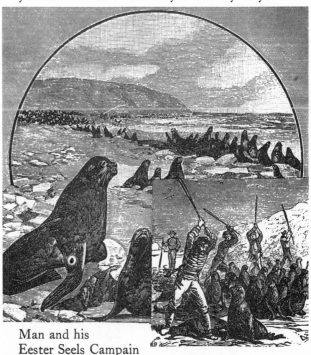

Man and his
Eester Seels Campain

Revolution. This exstink bizness happened before, ya know, and to bigger beasts than us, and with bigger bi-cupids. But yer youman don't need no enemas like that when he's got hisself to do the exstinktin'. They say it's a dog-eat-dog whirled, but by hinkus, I never yet seen a dog eatin' anuther dog. It's Man doin' it to Man, not to menshun what goes on inside yer Marriage Contrack for yer Holy Acrimony. It's time we reelized we're all stuck in the same club . . . before we start usin' it on each other.

CHAP SEVEN: YER JOLLYGEE

If we're gonna git down to rock bottoms with yer Jogfree, we gotta start first with Jollygee, because most of what seems to be going on in yer beds, when you gits rite down to it, is Rock.*

After yer Erth got blown offa yer Son and got cooled down a bit from a hot Glob, yer Erly Mass still felt purty ruff, even tho' it had a kinda glassy look like yer tippical Sardy nite drunk. There was no Notions at the time, neether yer Atlantick nor yer Specifick. Jist mostly molsen golden Lava.

But after all this vulcanizing, wich got yer Erth deeply bored, yer Rock come up between periods. Probly under pressyer from other Rocks in the same bed, it got forced up between the sheets, otherwise it coodn't get no stratus-faction.

I dunno how many peeriods makes a Eara er how many Earas make yer Eepock, but you can find out how old yer Rock is if you check yer Eepock-marks. Fer yer stratusfied rocks all got laid horezuntally, and it shows. Now yer Bible sez the hole rig took seven days, and yer Jollygee-whist clames it was more'n four billyun year, so I s'pose the anser lies in between as the fella said on his hunnymoon.

*ITCHY FEETSNOTE: My boy Orville agrees. He clects sertin kinds of Rock, mostly Micky Jaggy and his Running Stones.

CHAP EIGHT: YER ERLY DAZE (4 BILLYUN B.B.C.**)

You take your avrage Erth and yer deelin' with a Rocky mudball with water on the side; the hole thing circum-vented by Air (two parts of yer Hydro-gin, one part Ox-gin, add Nite-gin, ster'n serve at room tempachure) and hung together by yer Law of Gravelty, wich makes a whirl of a differnce. It was when yer Erth made water that all of a sudden it had a Notion, and that brake up some of yer rock into Sandy bottoms and the rest into continence.

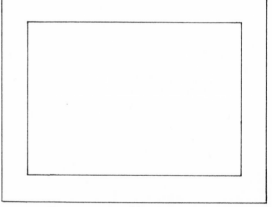

Air

Some of yer Rock got wore down till it become a little Bolder, and some of yer Bolder got shimmied into Pebble, and some of yer Pebble got worried into Sand. But then sometime yer Sand and yer Pebble wood git together, form yer Conglomerate, and go in the Gravel bizness. Then there was yer Rock under pressyure and in heat until it's bin thru the changes, what they call yer Meta-murphyic. We got a lotta that kind on our farm. It's considered gneiss, even tho' it comes from disturbed and twisted beds.

Nobody knows fer sure when life started up or what caused it, mebbe the heat, but it sure started with yer small scales. First sign of life come from one sell (wich lernt how to bifurkate itself and raze more

**MOLSEN FEETNOTE: Befoar Bubbels Coold.

sells). Funny to think how life starts with a single sell, and sometimes ends with it, too, in yer penitentsherry.

Yer first low-lifes was yer spunge, yer meeba, and other soft-bodied organasms. They lived mainly on yer plant life (and I don't mean punchin' a time clock from 9 to 5), wich at that time was all undersee, so that meel-time in them days was mostly dullse.

Things sturd up a bit with yer Murine Inverted Inebriates. That'd be a big word fer more big words . . . yer gastlypods, yer brackypods, and yer trilly-bites. What'sat all about? Algy. Now I know yer Algy is yer scum of yer Erth, jist lying around on stanknant water doin' nothin' but change the color of it. But it leads later on to yer snale and yer clam with mussels. And when the good Lord calls them all home, they go to make up yer Corl Reeths, wich is where all them retired fossils go to ther reward, much like yer Canadyan Sennet.

While all this was goin' on at yer mucky bottom, nothin' atall was shakin' up above yer water level, sept mebbe a few ferns wavin' and some mountin bilding by yer rolling stones. But by and by, yer seeweed become yer swamped grass and that give way to yer little Herb. Before you knew it, things was jumpin' with some bitsy insecks. Nobuddy knows where they come from 345 millyun yeers ago, but they bin back every summer since.

CHAP NINE: YER MESSY-ZOO-HICK

This is yer peeriod when a lotta animals dryed therselfs off. A lot of yer Marines that tried to come up on land and sun bath fur a spell ended up ex-stink on yer beech. But, after a time, a couple amp-fibbers develop what become AC-DC about yer land or sea. Mosta them went on to hire things, like climbin' trees, but a couple of them dubble-gated wet-or-drys is still around doin' ther crawl both places. Yer Terrypin is a turkle the size of a Folksywagen or a Toyola Coronary and was one of the first of yer bi-foke-alls to throw itself up on Terry Firmer and lay an aig. This last year I bin tryna order some of them things from Florider and breed 'em all winter. The wife she'd druther I breed topical fish, but I don't think I can stay under water that long.

Yer Messy-zoo-hick peeriod is divided into three subdivishuns (even in them days they made consessyuns). Yer Try-assid, yer Your-ass-hick, and yer Cretin-ages.

Try-assid: This was when life was found up a tree—and has bin purty much there ever since. Yer tree come in two tipes: yer decidyou-us, and yer undecidyous, the kind that woodn't make up its mind to be a Chrissmus tree er a big furn. Mosta

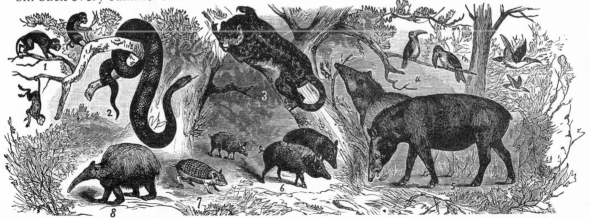

After yer evolootion   1. Simple Simions   2. Anna Conga   3. Jagger   4. Two-Can   5. Taperd
6. Peckery   7. Harmadildo   8. Aunt-Eater

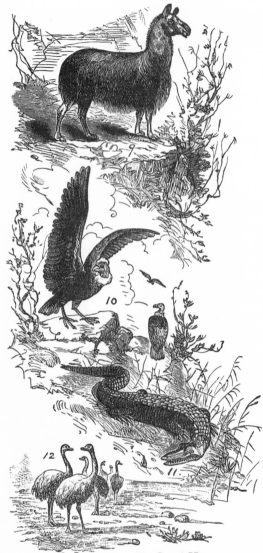

9. Lammer   10. Cond-Her
11. Crock Dial   12. Oster-rich

these erly trees becum carbon-snifferus, wich ment they went to the dogs and ended up a bit uminous in a cole-bin. Some of yer rocks took minrals and got on the Gold Standerd, wile others give in to pressure, cracked ther shales, and become oil.

Your-ass-hick: A old-time map of this second peeriod wood do no good, fer all yer mountin and valley, even yer lake and notion, was in differnt places, like in spring with the wife's livin' room fornitcher. Most of Yerp was water-log. The reesin

yer mounting was hire in places whur nowadaze you can't see none is on accounta like yer avrage harried and married man—they bin all ground down to stumps.

Cretin-ages: Only thing stickin' above water on our continence was yer Appleachin's. Yer Swish Alp was alreddy startin' to fold, and Mother Nature had not yet gotten her Rockies off. All this mountin bilding is called OROGENY by her later prodjenny but, since it still keeps changing, it's hard to keep tract of her Orogenous zone. At the end of this third peeriod, the three star s'lection wood have to be *cole*, *oil*, and yer *muskeeter*, wich should be Canda's nashnal Ember sted of yer Beever, if numbers means anything.* The only other flyin' thing round at the time was yer TERRY DUCKTAIL, a kind of ex-spear-mintal bird with no feathers. You'd wonder how the durn thing cud git offa the ground, and you'd think twice before sending anything with it air-male. It's now obscoleen and not herd.

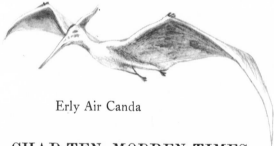

Erly Air Canda

CHAP TEN: MODREN TIMES

I'm talkin' bout the last 63 millyun years. We was finely gittin' our head above water, the mountins was unfolding as they shood, and our hole continence was startin' to shape up like yer Rammicknally on the wall or yer Funken Wagonall.

Mind, it were still No Man's Land. But them mammarals as hung around stopped livin' offa the sea and kep grazing more and more innards. And they was workin' ther way into bean more like we have now, instedda yer armor platers outa yer Flintstones Age. Coarse yer erly horse

*BIT FEETNOTE: A single skeeter lays 30 thou aigs a day, and there's no tellin how many a married one gits laid.

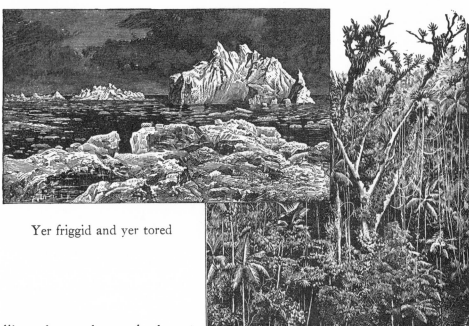

Yer friggid and yer tored

was still more like a dog, and yer erly dog was more like yer late-bloomin' pig. As for yer erly bird, it still got wurms. I gess some things hasn't changed since, o my goodness, Cretayshus times.

It was oney the last million year that we cud say Happy Berthday to Man, who finely dropped from yer top of the tree whur he'd bin co-rabbitin' with yer Gibberon and yer Orange-U-Tang. He sure picked a rotten time to git up offa his forepaws, fur he walked into the longest cold spell anybody's ever had, even incloodin' the one this last spring.

I dunno why they call yer Ice Age yer Plasterseen peeriod, becuz everything froze harder than last year's cow-pad. Mosta Yerp and Canda was blow zerode, more like that place wher they keep yer Suthern Pole, yer Aunt Article. In Canda, any yuman bean with enny git up and go got up and went. They crossed yer forty-ninth parrlel, never stopt til they come to Myammy Florider, and staid there, wether they was retired or not.

When yer Iced Age started, yer caved-in Man dint have two sticks to rub together. But he shore lerned fast and even invented how to speak langridge with his fulla man, on accounta everybody's teeth

was still shattering. Yer Meatier-ollygists say that yer Glassy Ears has bin defrostin' further'n further back up North ever since. But you cooda fooled me round some of my parts. I think yer Ice is comin' back fur to stay, becuz last year we even froze the Knockers off our big front door.

CHAP ELEVEN: YER ERTHY MOVEMINTS

Yer Erth may be yer deadbody, but by gol she's never still, fur she rolls over on her axes every 2–4 hours.* Did you know at the same time yer Moon is going round with yer Erth, yer Erth is too-timing by resolving to go around with her Son wunce a year?** (That'd be yer New Year's Revolootion.) This sorta thing is goin' on day and nite, which is why we're all of us

*COLD FEETSNOTE: The wife sez that's nothin' cumpaired with me, and she wants twin beds fer Chrissmus.

**INGROAN FEETNOTE: Sounds to me like incents.

goin' around haff lit. Wich means that one haff of yer whirled can't see how th'other haff lives.

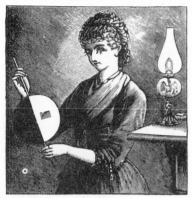

Haff lit

Sometime yer Erth has big tilts on her oar-bits, and this deet-ermins weather or not we're in season.

Yer Erth is divvied up into four Hemsfearoids, Norse and Souse fer yer Inseason and yer Out, East and West fer yer Grey Cup. Wich is why during yer Winter Solisitus, Eskymos go to bed with eech other fer six munths, while yer Argenteeny boppers stay up fer yer Carnal in Reo.

Long about yer Verminal Equalnots, they change sides, and then yer Eximoe is stayin' up all night huntin' bare, wile them Archintime grouchos is snoring among the Pampers.

CHAP TWELVE: HOW TO GIT A FIX

Yer Equador is the big bellyband acrost yer Erth's middle, and on eether side of her is yer markers fur the beginnings of yer Termpermint Zone, on our side yer Topical Canso, and on them others yer Pappycorn. These two Mane Topics of Conservation is also Parrlells of Lassitude on the side. There's more parrlells of Lassitude than you can shake yer Sextint at, every one of them depending frum yer Equador at a differnt angl of dangl.

Slicing the other way down yer Pole is

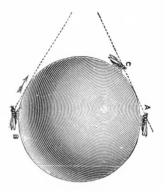

Time—as yer froot flies

yer Parrlells of Lunge-tude. Insted of mezzuring off from yer bellyband, them up-and-down fellas starts from yer PriMer Ribbyon, wich is tied up in the Mean Time with yer Jolly GreenWitch of England.

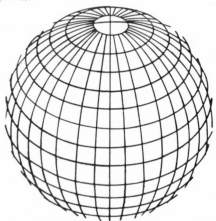

Wirld colander fer time keeping

When yer Lunge-tudes inter-sex with yer Lassetudes, that's when yer Erth's a netball fulla grids . . . but don't ask me hominy grids in yer Murkeater's Perjection.

Yer PriMer Ribbyon is not only good fer finding yer wearabouts, speshully if you live in Greenwitch, but it gits the hole whirled wound up with yer Standerd Times.*

Them as nose say the only acrid way of telling yer exack creek time is to have a

*MARKTIME FEETNOTE: I don't mean them two noospapers they have over there. I mean the strokes give off by Big Benz near yer West Minister's Abie.

Son Dile. By swinjer, what'll they think of next! (Wonder if they've broke it to John Cameroon Swayznee with his strapping Timax?) Accordion to this noofangled Solar timepees, Tronto peeple is two minutes differnt from yer foke on th'other side of the mountin in Humiltin. Trubble with Trawntuh peeples is they haven't got no time fur peeple in Humultun ennyways, sept when ther Aggernuts and them Pussycuts meat in ther Cups at yer I-Never-Winn Stadyum.

Yer Dating Game: When yer Green Witch has gone about as fur as she can go in yer Meantime, she finely bumps in the middle of yer Specifick Ocean into yer Date line.* This gits purty tecknickle, but the upshat of it all is that if you folla the advice of Horse Greeley and keep on moving west, by the time you git to yer High-weigh-in Ilands, er even up north Alasker with yer Illusions, you lose a hole day. But, by gol, every well hung-over travellin' man knows that.

*HEATNOTE: We has the same trubble with young Orville on our party line.

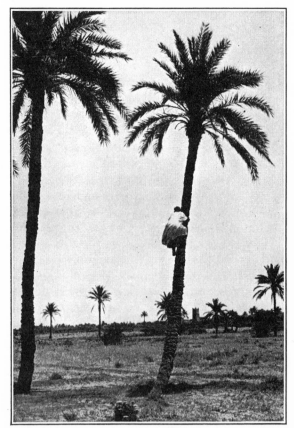

Checking dates

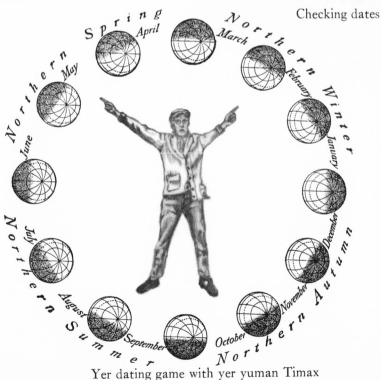

Yer dating game with yer yuman Timax

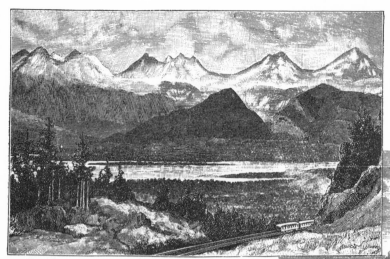

Before—

—and after the passage
of yer wind

CHAP THIRTEEN: AT THE MERSEY OF YER ELFENTS

Now wen they say elfents, they don't mean them big patchy dermis with the gray wrinkled soots that look like a big Folkswagen you can't tell wich end has got the trunk and wich the drive-shaft. Yer elfents of Jogfree that we're at the Mersey of is jist the same things make us frustrate every day . . . yer wind, yer wether, and yer tide, wich don't wait up fer no man.

Wether: As yer Erth terns, yer Atmossfear gose along with it. Beyond the behind of that is yer Strutsfear, wich don't have no wether at all but other problems fer Assternuts, sich as witlessness. But it's yer Atmossfear that sets the tone of the place and brings on yer climaxtick conditions like clowds, both yer Accumulus, Sirrius, and yer Nimphus.

Yer clime-it reely depend on three things: yer tempachure, yer wetness, and yer wind.

Yer Wind: Biggest of all is yer wind, wich is a peece of air on its way sumplace elts. When the wind moves up yer cold parts from yer hot ones, it's on accounta hot air rises to fill up the Vackyume (speshully at 'lection time). Mother Nature abwhores them Vackyumes and it behoovers her to fill it up with somethin' else.*

Yer avrage wind is not too vylent, jist goin' from yer high to yer low, that's how they blow, more of a ventlater than a vyalater. If she gits heated, we git a rise out of her. And when she gits offal high, she'll fall back on yer Erth in the form of perticipation (wich is CBC fer rain).

Rain is jist wind havin the vapors, feeling dense, gittin dropsy, and bringin mebbe also snow er sleet er even the hale with it.

Another kind of wethering done by yer wind is jist waring down yer mountings

*SUCKING FEETNOTE: The wife agrees, speshully when the thing backs up and splits her bag.

till she's sandpapered smooth as a baby's butte. But don't count on it rite away . . . takes ten thou year fer to eeroad away three inch. Sounds like a guvmint project, don't it? Sure wish the Galumphing Inflammation had the same rate.*

Yer Wet: Why don't no rain fall on yer desserts? Well sir, as you pass yer wind from yer friggid zones to yer hot spots, yer vapors git so absorbed that yer wind seems to be able to hold it till it gits past yer dry townships and drops on to yer wets. And that's what causes Local Opshun.

Yer Air: Everyone is livin' under pressyure these days, but if they new how much they'd have a shag fit. Not so much yer bird of pray on clowd nine, but us poor immorals down blow. You kin check yer Gage after, but I'm tellin' you she's up to fifteen pound fer every one of yer square's inch. You take yer average square incher like myself, I got 30,000 pounds of air on top of me (plus the secund morgidge).

But if we wasn't fulla it, yer Air, we'd be crushed flattern'n a pee on a platter. So be careful you don't let off too much

*TIED FEETNOTE: No thanks to Pearl Bumtree, yer Fud Prices Revue Broad.

steem or you'll end up thinner than yer Erodedendron in yer Family Bible.

Yer Tide: It's the Moon working nites and using pull on yer Erth. Never mind yer Artick Power, this Tide stuff is outa this wurld. It wurks in all tempacheers of water. And since yer Erth is more'n three quarts water (like yer skimmy milk), the Moon pulls on them beeches like a big maggot with the arn file-ings. And yer pull is dubbled up when the Son gits on the same side, and you git a rip-off tide can suck youse under quicker'n a jackass-rabbit movin' thru Scotch thissle. Them Spring rip-tides do a lotta damnage, like turnin' young men fancy instead of studding fer ther exams. And if you're a Weerd Wolf like Lawn Shaney, you gits hair in the pam of yer shoulders.

No wonder them old-timers in Grease used to warship yer Moon with a pull like that. That's why they figgered she had a bo and arras, and they called her Diana Sweets, yer Hunterass.**

**SWEETS FEETNOTE: Her fella Gods on Mount Limpus, who folleyed all her movemints, called her Girt with a Quiver.

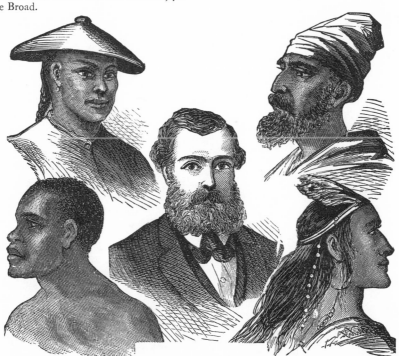

Kernel Sanders' Branch Offisers

Yer Commnest Fackter: Man has put Mother Erth thru the changes more'n anybody. He sure has bin a fast wurker tamperin' with his Mother's Naycher. I don't meen the furst millyun years. I mean jist the last fifty. If my Grate Grampa Farquharson cood see what has happint to the old Homestud, he'd rotate in his beer. Mosta his hardwood bush has bin cut off, feelds that was furtle is now barn, and by barn I don't mean the place whur the stock do their Animal Husbandry. I mean barn where nothin' grows on accounta yer leaches in yer soil and yer leeches at the Bank.

When Grate Gramp come over from County Furmanna as an Ulcer imgorant, our hole districk was what they call yer Prime Evil Willternest, give er take a few lumbering setlers. Well sir, yer Willternest is gone now, but seems to me we got more Prime Evils than ever. Oh, we ain't the first to have done this. Yer Roamin' Umpires they done a bang-up job of explorting ther own penisula and finely putting the boot to it. Yer Spainyards they had a bit more sents. They explorted overseize and put the gold blocks to yer Inkys and yer Asstex.

We done the same with our own Injians by snuffling off ther Bufflo. Insted of puttin' a fence around them with reservations, we dun that insted to th'Injuns.

And now them City Oil slickers is starting to work on the parts of the Whirled wich is so far uninhibitable. And if it ain't them, it's yer Atomical Bums testing us on their Specifick Atholes and spraying the air with Playhouse 90 till we're all in danger of Falloff.

I'm afrayed yer Man fackter is yer main fackter. And we're all gonna have to quit if he don't.

Part Two: Yer Parts

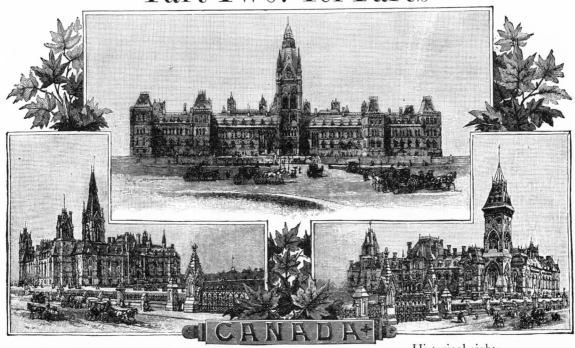

Histerical sights

CHAP FOURTEEN: CANDA: YER OVERALLS VIEW

To most of yer whirled Canda is mostly froze waist. They mite be s'prised to know we got some cackus* plants in Elberta and pam trees in the lobbly of yer Impress Hotel in Victeroria.**

Wether er not yer Chinee er yer Texassan admit it, Canda is yer second bigst place on Erth, give er take yer Serviet Roosia. She's as long as she's abroad, from Ellensmear Ile in yer hardend Articks to yer murkry bottoms of Lake Eery, from Vancoover's Iland wher they keep yer penshners to yer Noofy Saint's John wher they keep yer ambulents.

Fizzyoggerfee: This vast, scrawling land was spewked out of yer Erth's pasteerior in molson form and bilt up over yer neons by steddy stresses and stranes. She's bin tilt, twist, crunched togither, renched a part, and genrully shattered on . . . much like yer avrage marridge.

Canda: Frum Scratch
Canda started between yer icy sheets from scratch and has the marks to prove it. It was from them glassy ears sneakin' back into cold storge and tearin' yer bedrock. And who nose if they ain't on ther way back? After the way spring come along this year long after yer Verminal Equalnuts, I don't think our Joon bugs showed up till after thrashin' time.

After we got defrosted, we discovered yer Erth has a lotta crust and we got the hardist parts. If youse have ever tried to plow yer pre-Crambian Sheeld, you'll reelize it'll take a lot before this country splits up.

I dunno why we worry about our Unititty so much. Last year it was the turn of yer Alberta Seprators*** to say they was

*PARTY FEETNOTE: Yer cackus is not to be confused with yer cockus, wich is p'litical. In a cackus, the pricks is on th'outside.

**OLD PARTY FEETNOTE: Them pams is pottied like mosta yer gests.

***DIVIDED FEETNOTE: We got one in our creem shed. Never give us enny trubble at all.

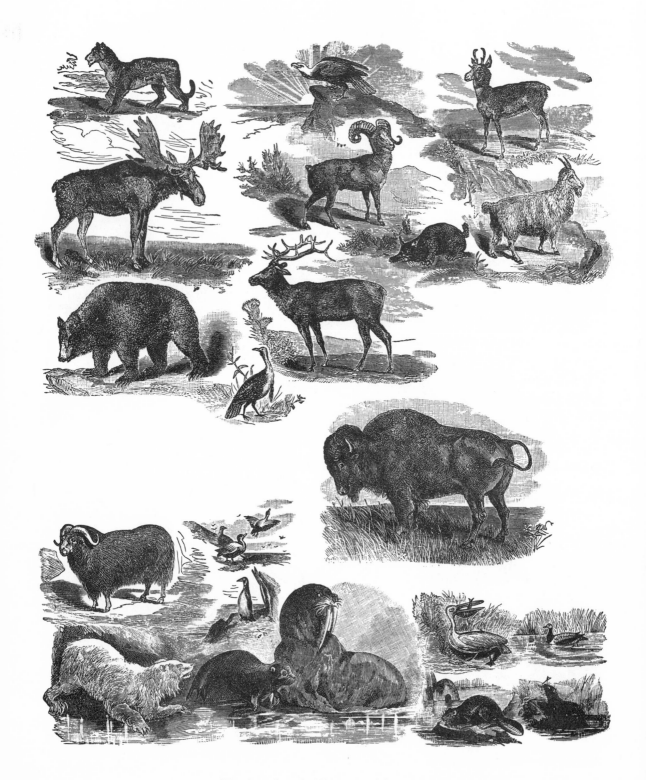

Natchuralized inhibitants of Canda

gonna defecate from the rast of us. But as of Jooly one, we're headin' fer a hundert and ate in the shade and still alive and kickin' (and screemin' at eech other). It's the differnces we got what keep us together (that and everybuddy hatin' yer Air Canda cawfee). But everybuddy in this land has allus been purty pukewarm about all the other parts, sept in November when ther in ther Gray Cups. I think we'll be all right so long as we keep a good gripe on arselves.

CHAP FIFTEEN: CLIMAXTICK CONDISHUNS

This chapter of Mr. Farquharson's book has been censored. Gage Publishing has never seen such language.

The Editor

Well I'll be a brass munky! Balled out by my edter! What does he noe about cold—he spends the winter in his West Undys.

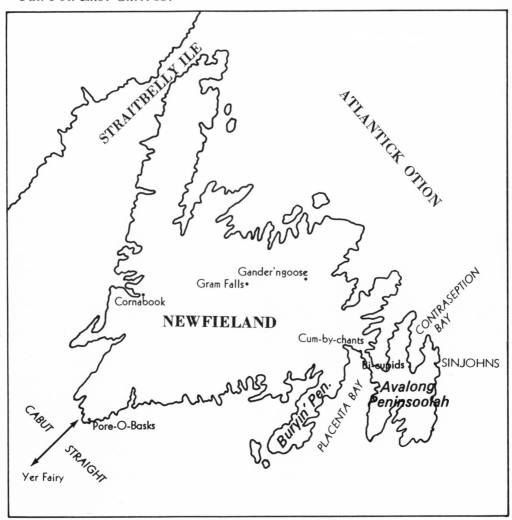

Newfyland

NEWFIELAND: GAITPOST TO YER FAR EEST

This must be yer most flu-over place on erth. It's on yer Grate Circus root fer mosta yer arelines, incluedin yer Pannedamurricans. It's a shame peeple never stop to take more'n a Gander at the place, fer yer Newfy is no joke. That don't meen they don't have no sense of humor, fer they look at life with a cod's tung in ther cheek. These peeple is no squares. They've bin all round yer cirkle, inports and out, and thru all ther trubbles they kin cum up from a tickle with a twinkie in ther eye, after jigglin' ther squids.

It's ironickle that yer Newfy at 25 yeer old is still yer Noo Canadyun,* becuz they was sure yer first to settle down.

Histerically speekin', it'd be yer 1610 that a buncha Micksed Irish and Angled Sacksons was brung out by some Guy from Bristle and bogged all down together at a place called Cupids. It was later changed to Bi-cupids, fer to git Irishmen and Anglishmen to live togither without splittin' is like pulling teeth. They're still havin' fites every Sardy nite sints 1610,** jist two year after yer French connection

*DIFFICULT FEETNOTE: That'd be in '49 when Joey led them into the big time outa yer small woods.

**TIMELY FEETNOTE: Ten after four.

was foundered at Cue-bec by Sam the Sham-plane.

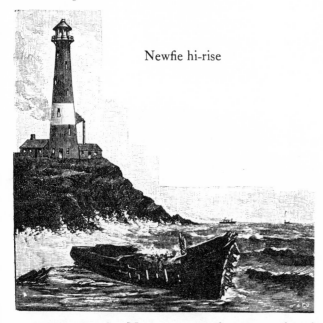

Newfie hi-rise

Aggercultyer: Not too much aggercultyerin' in Newfyland. Jist a short stretch in yer Avalong Penisyouliar. Yer West parts is fulla mountains what has bin wore-down and wore-out by yer erogenous zones, but peeple live mainly on their outpores. Leese they did, till Joey Smallswood moved them to yer imports fer to be members of his Well-fare Estate. Some peeple think by gittin' them outa the boats and into the facktrees he turned out to be no more'n a little ship disturber.

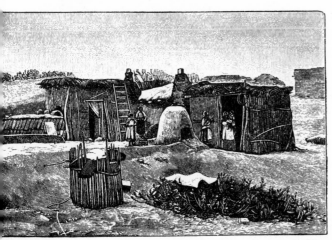

Outport houses

Yer Froot: Berryin' is big in Newfieland. I don't meen funereals. I mean yer razz and yer straw and yer cran and yer blew. They used to stop yer train, the Bull-it, so's the local rakes cud git ther cans full. It seems berrys grow partickler good on burnt-up land, wich probly makes fer more arson around than nessry.

Yer Hunt: Moose is big, too. Everybody is alweez after a little country meet, and cum Eester time they don't give the kids rabbids er seels. Yer Newfieland kid is more'n likely to git a choclit moose.*

Yer Fur: I think the only trappers wud be yer lobsterers, but there's a lotta breeding in and out of yer fur-boring animals. Used to be foxing, but now it's mostly minking sentered around yer Dildo. Seems they raze mink stoles cuz the wimmen don't have the eyes fer yer foxfers no more.

Yer Mine: Yer minral-oilogists is still sinkin' ther drills looking fer ther own loob jobs. In the meentime Long Pawn has a talc mine wich grinds out baby's powder. But I think yer Newfies are gitting sick of talc, talc, talc, and want a little action.

Speekin' of sick, that's nuthin' to what goes on in yer Buryin'Penancesular. That's where minors bring up yer Fluorspar fer to help make stainliss steal. Don't help them minors too much tho'. They gits stains on ther buckin' bronckial toobs from all that ultra-violents. And they can't seem to git much of a move outa yer Workmen's Constipation Bored, even when they sing them that song "The Boys from Impfazeema."**

I think the owners is satisfied with this nifty fifty-fifty derangement: they keeps the ore, and the minors gits the shaft.

*HOT FEETNOTE: They got big horns and they must be hard to hold when they dip them big things in yer bilin' hot choclit!

**SORE FEETNOTE: First line is "I's the bye that gits the troat."

Yer Murine Life: A safer way of makin' a livin' (active without bein' too radio) is goin' down to the shore and takin' in yer Irish moss. Old timers still likes to gather ther moss, but the yung prefurs to stay home and lissen to yer Rolling Stones. They say they'd be in big bizness if you could perklate that moss into Irsh Cawfee.

But it's the fishin' is still yer mane drag. You give a Newfylander sumthin' on the end of his line, he'll show you he's a master baiter. A lotta then gits cricket-sized long about Eester Seels time, fer goin' out on th'ice and puppin' them lil aminals off fer to make club sammitches, er seel-flipped-over-pie. They beet up on them the way the rest of yer NH Hellers treets yer Loss Angles Golden Seels. But if yer Newfylanders stopped seeling, there'd still be lots of Scandlenavyans and Porchgeese come all the way from yer A-sores. It'd take a wale of a embargo fer to stop yer slotter now.

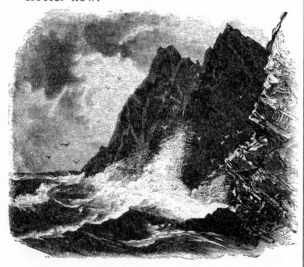

Quiet day in Newfie

Yer Captoll: I fergot to menshun Saint's John, a perl of a harbor, deep, rumey, and easy to enter . . . jist like the lady of ex-peerients she is.

Yer Wether: Some peeple think Newfie-landers goes round in a perpetchul fog. That's only cuz they is cot midstreem between yer Labbydoor currant comin' down from Forlorn Greeneland and yer Golf streem, the well-known water inter-corse from Florider. These two streems meet jist like the two laigs of a pair of pants, and there is Newfyland stuck in the crutch of the sityation. And when yer warm air hits yer friggid, there's nothin' much to do but sit around and duck the fog.

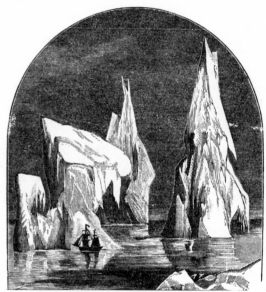

Ice flows in Sin Jawn harber

Yer Ile: First drill seshuns lookt good, but the Shaheen has gone off by now. Still pumping up and down at Contraception Bay.*

*CHANGED FEETNOTE: Used to be called Cum-by-Chants B.P. (Before yer Pill).

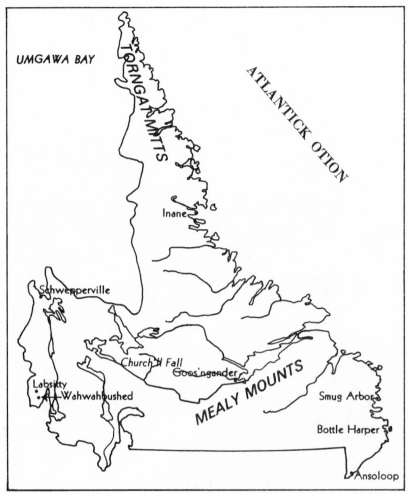

UMGAWA BAY

TORNGAT MTTS

ATLANTICK OTION

Inane

Schwepperville

Church'll Fall

Goos'ngander

MEALY MOUNTS

Labsitty

Wahwahbushed

Smug Arbor

Bottle Harper

Ansoloop

Labbydoor

YER LABBYDOOR

Looks purty rocky but, in fack, was settled down before any of us come along, when yer Viking took a liking. Next come yer German Method Mishnarys. (I s'pose yer heethen Viking musta cleer out when he found yer Mishyuns Impossible.) Mind you, speekin' of that, there arn't no roads to speek of even to-day, and the only way to set foot in to yer inteerier is to rail at Cuebeck (wich is wot Newfieland has bin doin' ever since the Yanks uncovert yer arn ore). Both sides clames "Yer mine! Yer mine!", but ackshully the mine b'longs to yer Amurrican investered intrusts who moved in erly to sit on one of the whirld's biggest orehouses.

There's so darn much of the stuff it jist lies round on top of yer ground, up Schlepperville way. And all the diggers hasta do is what they call yer open-pits mining. (Orville thinks that meens working with yer shirt off.)

But Labbydoorians is still singing the Wabush Blooze, on accounta that injurious-dickonal fite 'tween Newfy and Cue-beck. It seems the mines are in yer Newfy sexion, and the ports (like Set Eeels) is in yer French parts. And the law says you can't de-ore arn into steal inside

of Labbydoor. (They probly smuggle it
out first-class air-male to the States.) But
till yer Newfs and yer Cube-beckers sort
that one out, they're gonna be morer less
on the horns of an enemma.

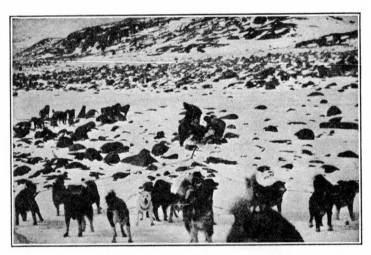

Lab dogs

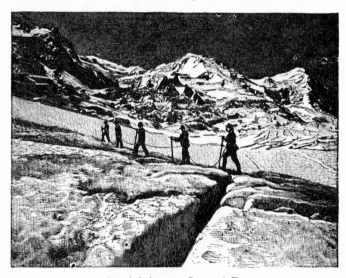

Deplaining at Goosed Bay

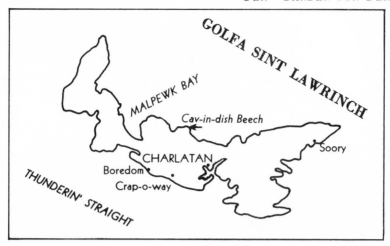

P.I.E.

YER P.I.E.

Is also called yer "Garden for yer Golf," on accounta all you can see on yer North shore is Merken tooriests down on ther hands and neeze lookin' fer a white dot in a cow-pad. They come from all over yer States with ther club bags and tee-caddies jist fer to have a few strokes. (Myself, I wun't know wich end of the caddy to grab aholt of. I think the only two good balls I ever hit was the day I stept on the garden rake by mistake.)

P.I.E. used to be a big pertater and corn center, "the eyes and ears of Canda," but I think the mane bizness of that lil Iland must be yer Tooriests now. It's becum so darn poplar a place that the most sot fer sooveneers is now peeces of P.I.E. itself. So yer Pervinshuls are startin' to say that furners from yer U.S. and Uppity Canada can't own no more land (speshully them North Shore sunsy beetches). Rite now they're tryna make it stick by passing a movement on the floor of ther lokal Common House. (That's where we started yer first Conflergration in 1864, 9 year before even yer Ilander was reddy to Conflerg.)

It ain't bin deesided as yit by her Sperm Cort, but yer Charlatans is alreddy got this noo law writ down in ther own Dunesday Book. I don't blame them too much

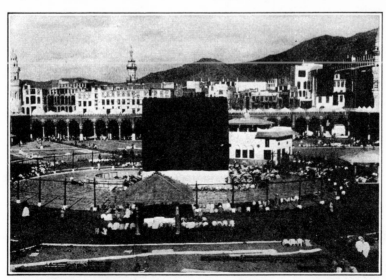

P.I.E. —Mecca of tworists

fer tryna keep private parts offa Rusty-cove and Cave-in-dish, fur I think every-buddy in yer John Q. Pubic shud be able to share ther sandy bottoms.

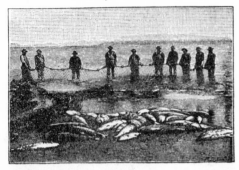

Beech party—sept fer the poor fish

The Injian name fer P.I.E. is ABIG-WAIT, wich is sort of a Mixmash word meenin' "Curdled by the waves." But most outlanders think it refurs to all the time you have to spend waitin' in line fer Fairies at Boredom or Cape Tormentintime.

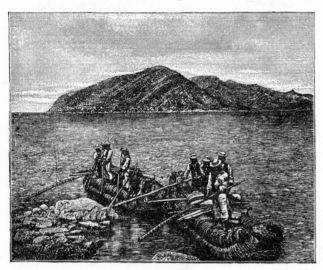

P.I.E. —Ferryland

The wife and I was down one year with the trots. (Valeda, she'd go anywares fer to sulk. Sez you can't git much closer to yer horse than that.) It was durin' yer Old Homes Week, and, my gol, they sure do got a lotta them around. I s'pose our own homested is purty run-down, too, but we don't go celibatin' it.

We was took around fer to see them tendin' ther taters up Crap-o way. (I think it's called that on accounta the prices they're gittin' fer 'taters. Makes them wonder what's a tuber for?) The nashnul antrim of P.I.E. is "Butt the Spud," wich is sung by Stumpin' Tom Cobley wile bangin' his board.

Mosta yer fishin' nowadaze is done by furners. Even Yerpeens come all the way over in ther Hunky dorys. Used to be yer P.I.E. catch was wholey mackrel, but evry summer now they have a contest fer to "Mame that Toona." We was took out to yer East End, to Soory, fer to watch yer lokels settin' on ther lobster pots,* then up the other end bobbin' fer oyster in yer Malpewk Bay.

At nite we was took in by yer Charlatan's Fester-all at the Conflagellation Senter fer to see a show they got up on the platform called yer "Lil Orphan Annie of yer Green Gages" (bout a girl who et so much raw froot her hair turned the same culler). The nite we was ther, one a the acters, Matthew, had a gas attack and never cum back. I think myself he was jist plain embarsed havin' to sing "Annie Green Gages *never* change". . . wich, speshully in the summer-time, don't sound too san-terry.

Mind you, yer P.I.E.landers don't change too much. They are still nice, shy and preserved, and accordion to yer statis-ticleticks, they're the only pervinshuls what has less peeple today than a hundert year ago. And that's jist good manors, not bean on the pill er havin' vasillectummys.**

Jist before we left yer P.I.E.land, I ast one farmer hard by Kapok Beech jist what he was gonna do if he wasn't aloud to sell his land to some furner from Trawnto. He figgered he wud start razin' yer Terrypin. Now yer Terrypin is them big turkles from Florider, 'bout the size of a Folksy-wagon

---

*CLAWD FEETNOTE: The wife thinks them Marim-tiders is offal clever fer to train a lobster to sit on a pot.

**INTUMATE FEETNOTE: Yer vasillectummy is what most yung cupples has today when they announces that ther thinkin' of tyin' the knot.

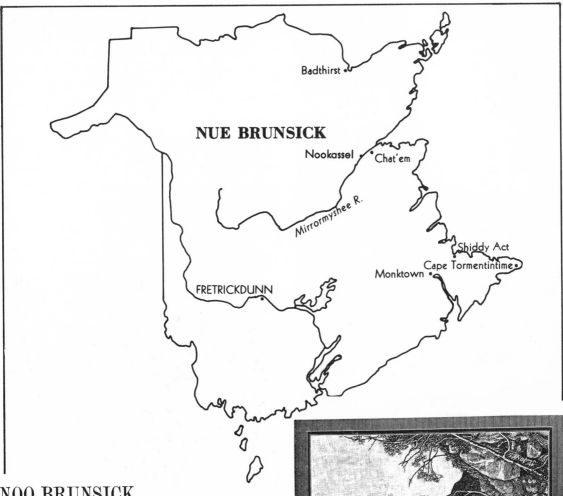

NUE BRUNSICK

Badthirst

Nookassel · Chat'em

Mirrormyshee R.

Shiddy Act
Cape Tormentintime ·
Monktown ·

FRETRICKDUNN

NOO BRUNSICK

Yer Land of Wooden Water is so-called on accounta it has the most lumbring of yer Marmtiders, along with the biggest swells from yer Tide. Yer Tide-wash cum in twice a day, even Sundys and holdaze, during yer Tooriest seezin. Say what you like, but yer Noo Brunsicker has got the fastest rizing water in the world... comes rite up yer PettycoatAct and bores them twice a day. They even got a Titled Bore, probly named after one a yer Loylist flounderers what excaped from yer Republican Demmycrats in '76. And yer capitalist city, Sinjon, has so much Tide in its narra gorge that it has a back-up falls that re-gorge-itates itself at this end of yer Loylist Tail. If Nagger Falls cud do that, ther'd be no falling off of Tooryists.

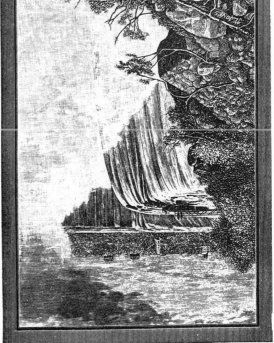

sllaF desreveR

Noo Brunsick is not too much fer yer urbanes. It goes in more fer yer dense roorals. That's becuzz the biggest industree is yer tree. All ya have to do is watch 'em grow and cut 'em down . . . that's what they call a life of yer natcheral vegetatin'.

But, if prest, Noo Brunsickers can turn ther hand to anything, fer ther used to gittin' the back of evrybuddy else's hand . . . that's how prest they've bin. They kin make anything from mops and brumes at yer Landcaster brush works* to Fiddleheds fer sympathy orchesters.

One thing they've bin able to raze besides forsts is rich men. You take yer Max Aching, who went over to Angland and

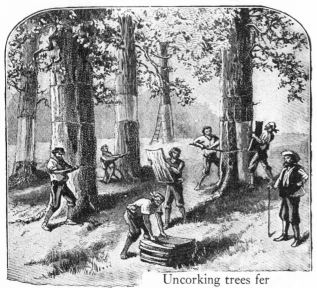

Uncorking trees fer
to git shuggered off

sold newspapers till he becum Lord High Beever's Book, and spent the rest of his time in London keeping up ther Evening's Standerds. You take yer Sir Jim Dunn, who give so much of his munny back to Fredstrictin that they din't feel so bad Dunn by. And last but not leese in yer accounts, you take yer Casey Irving (before he takes you). He's the fella what invented that game, Monopply, and he's now restin' down there on his Bannanas.

*FURRY FEETNOTE: Noo Brunsickers clames they lerned from us Uppity Canadians how to give everybuddy the brush.

But, my gol, if they export mosta ther rich in Noo Brunsick, that still leeves an offal lot more pore. Some Noo Brunsickers live on yer sub-sistems level waitin' fer a sud-sidy. I mind the time Pry Mister Terdo cut off ther Winter Werks pogrom jist becuz his Minster of Infernal Revenoors, Edgar Bergen . . . I think that's the name . . . the fella who coodn't keep his pipe lit and yet told the rest of us how to mind our fiskal affairs . . . told Terdo it wud help the inflammation to have a little of yer unemployablemint. By now everybuddy up in Ottawa reelizes that Unemploymint isn't Working. But that gallumphing inflammation is goin' ahed like a forst fire.

There's fishin' here in yer Middle Eest, mostly dun by toorists round yer Pastmyquota Bay. The Murkins come up and all they wants is yer trout, nothin' but the trout. Can't unnerstand why they leave the Rest-to-goose sammon. Yer locals do a little weerd fishing, but there's some sane ones as well. Some of the old-timers still goes in fer sord fishing, but myself I preefur yer rod and yer reel. Or specktater sports like yer ShiddyAct Lobster Festerall.

Some of them on yer Fundy-side of the Streem clames they makes munny scallopin', altho' I bet not as much as them ones that stand outside yer Maybeleeve Gardens during yer Stanley's Cups.

One thing honorably menshunable is yer Noo Brunsick candy. They sure rung the Ganong with them, Moir less. And it's hard to beet yer Mirrormyshee blewberries. The place is fulla pickers, wich is handy, fer after ours they love to shake a boot with some country music with a little western sangwidged in.

Noo Brunsickers has eyes fur ptaters, too; they bug them more'n yer P.I.E.s. A lotta farmers is still bying yer D.D. and T. on the side so's they can drop a little aphid. Mosta yer ptaters that is not et is alloud to go to seed, sept fer those sent to yer St. Hubert barbecue in Cue-bec fer to keep them in the chips.

Don't git th' idee that there's nuthin' goin' on in yer town-life. You take yer Monktown now. It's a big raleway junkshun point, and everything comes together in yer Hump yard (speshully after dark). It's got a Maggotnetick Hill that gives New Brunsickers the optickle deluzin that ther gettin' sumplace when they reely arn't. Monktown's also the place has got yer only Interdependent M.P. fer the Common House, becuz Bob Stansfeeld had sich a hard time keepin' up with the Joneses boy. It seems the Monktown peeple exercised ther french-fries fer yer one-lingamilism, so they won't have to have no "flock-on demaze" on ther cornflakes boxes.

I dunno what yer French is s'posed to do livin' up there on ther Bathurst streets. Mebbe they'll all git sint to Noorleens like that pore girl Evasseleen and her Royl Arcadians three hunnert yeers ago. My gol, if we all has to go back whur we first cum from, that meens even yer Mixmax Injians will end up hard by Mongrowlia in yer Go-bye Dessert. Serch me where yer Jones famly comes from(sounds to me like a name a fella makes up when he wants to be a sneek in a motel). But if they like jist the one langwidge, mebbe they should move to Cue-beck now that Premeer Boracic has give them Westmounters a hedache with his Bill 222.

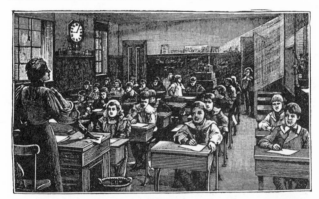

Before —

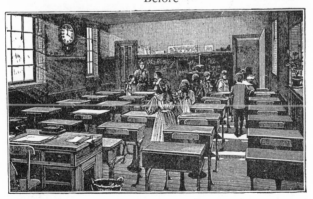

— and after yer 222

CUEBEC:
LA BILL PRO-VAUNCE

Bilingamal Innerductshun:

Mesdames et messoeurs
Jimmy suis appel Charolais
Farqueueharson
Et je suis heureux d'ecrire de sez
affaires . . .

My ladees and my sisters
My name is Charlie Farquharson and
I squeeze my own apples.
And I'd be happy at this stage of
my creer to have 16 affairs.

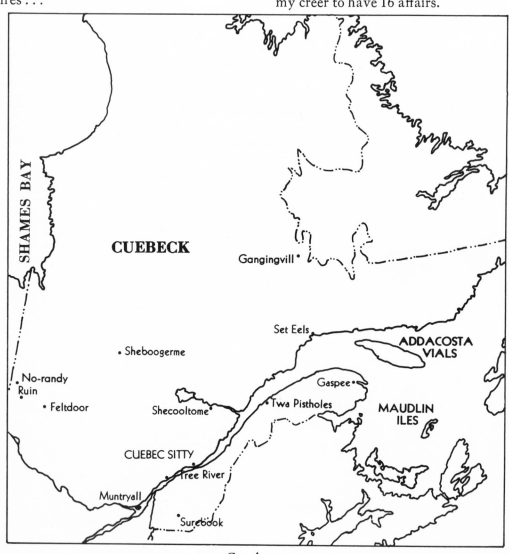

SHAMES BAY

CUEBECK

Gangingvill

Set Eels

ADDACOSTA
VIALS

• Sheboogerme

No-randy
Ruin

Gaspee

• Feltdoor

Shecooltome

Twa Pistholes

MAUDLIN
ILES

CUEBEC SITTY

Tree River

Muntryall

Surebook

Cue-bec

Cue-beck is an old Algonk-you-win word meening "it gits narrerer here." But that was the old-time place before yer Quiet Riot Rebelyoution, leading up to them Exposing therselves in '67.

La Climate: In one French word...FREUD

La Land: When it comes to farmin', yer French is basecally strippers. I don't meen like yer Dookybores. I'm talking about

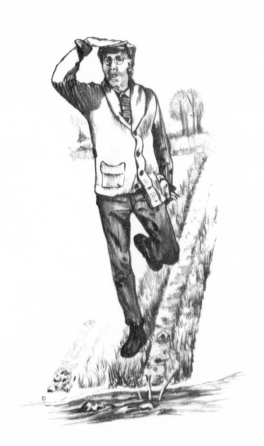

"Some jour, Orville, toot this will be votres."

the way of passing on the old place, wich is by terring a strip offa the old man's. In them old days, everybuddy lived offa yer seenery. I don't meen a place that's nice to look at, like yer Rich Loo Valley. I meen yer farm was owned by the oldest man in the family, one of yer seenery sittizens, and when he passed over, his land was passed around to all them sons. And you know there'd be plenty of them, becuz even to day yer French is never too strong on berth controll, relying more on yer sense of natteral rhithm (noan as Vaticacan Ruelet).

Now yer old-time Pee-super he thot land was no good less it fronted on yer water. (Them strangers what bin comin' up to our Muskoker fer the past 35 yeers thinks the same way.) In them daze, land wern't no good less it was on the river, on accounta it was purty near yer only loco-meens a motion. So when the land was divvied up every time yer generation went over the Gap, yer average seenery ended divvied like so many bolling allys.

And that's what's eetin' yer next gen-ration of Cue-beckers. They're jist afraid they won't have a laig to stand on.

Lays Sitties: They don't look much diff-ernt from ars . . . sept fer jist yer sines everywears like *Defence de Fume* and *Icky Radio Canada*. In the countryside of yer Gaspy or yer Sagginany, you can sure tell it's Cuebeck by them Crucial-fixes by the side of the road. Or even one of them old drive-in ovens, becuz you take yer French they always got time by the side of the rode fer a little oven.

But in ther sitties you couldn't tell the differnts from us Angled Sacksons sept mebbe the langrige and the gud fud.

Muntry-All: You take yer Placed Darts. They got a restrunt there with more'n seventeen kinds of Excargo. You take yer excargo before it comes out of its shell—that'd be yer sluggy snale—but the way they down it up pipping hot in spicy Gaelic is downrite suckyouLent. (I jist has a bit of trubble gitting down the shells.)

Yer Calorie stampede ain't out West. It's here in Muntry-all, wether its yer Saint Hoobert Barby-queue, yer Gray None Snac Bar, er yer Holy Family re-strunt, 'pending on yer stayshun in life. And after dinner youse can bounce acrost the hole sitty on yer Metrow, wich has got inflatable tires to go with the prices. And they got fancy muriels to look at, even in yer uriels. And if you wanta git up above it all, you takes yer Otto-root to yer Lower-wrenchin Mountings. Yer Muntry-all Otto-root, that's the Cue-bec version of yer Nashnul Lottery.

Cuebec Sitty: Shood be seen in winter when everybuddy feels Bon Ami Carnal-vall . . . wich is French fer "I'm giving up after Lent." It's frendly fer a walled-in town. But it's a class place, divided in-to yer Uppers and Lowers with a big rock in between like yer Jibber-altar. Mosta

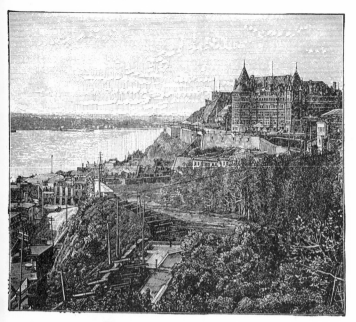

Uptown and downtown Cuebec

yer ackshuns happen around yer Placcid Arms in the Shadow of yer Frontknack. But the Cittydell lites up two times a yeer when its inhibited by yer Governing Genral. It was at yer Cittydell wher King Mackenzie met Rosyfelt and Winsome Churchle and confurred about yer Second Front (yer boarder between Ontaryo and Cuebeck). Funny thing, Cuebeck is yer largesse provence, and yet there's reely only a pair of big sitties. The rest is peeteeter as they say in yer buy-lingamal. Yer Valcoor is a small place, yet it has Bumbarded the rest of the hole contnint with Schmoe-mobeels. I figger we got next door to us on eyther side (between the 9th and 10th lines on yer forth concussion) mebbe 23 Skidoo.

Tree River is jist what it's name says… the place wher they chop off yer lims and roll 'em to a pulp. Twa Pisthole must be the place wher they make rest-rooms. They got more Saint places than you can ring around a rosery. St. Louis de Ha Ha was named after one who was tickled pink. Up in yer Shames Bay arear, they got a bran new place, St. Pollute du Lac.

Closet thing to Ottawa that Cuebeckers got is Hull … wich is wher yer Guvmint gose to drink ("I'll see ya in Hull first").

Hull is the home of yer matchless E.B. Eddy Cumpny, and was the inspirtration fer Bob Dillyun when he was playing at yer Tarts Senter acrost the river and writ that song "Yer Answer is Blowin' in the Wind."

Cuebeckers go in more fer big britch work than big towns … they got yer Muntryall Samplane, yer Jack Carter, and yer Cue-beck Cantreeleever Suspants Britch.

Mebbe on accounta all ther trubbled waters, Cuebeck is called "yer curdle of Noo France." It's also called La Bill Provaunce since Premeer Booracic went aginst our mygrain with his 222. That's the Bill that says you can go to the scool of yer choice s'long as you speek wot yer tolled. For eggsample, if you was Eyetalian and was let into Canda by yer Minster of Imgorance, Robert Android,* you have to give up the "fungoo Eetaliano" and start to "parley voo le madmoselle with Armenteers." Booracic figgers that yer Roman wasn't well-bilt in a day but, as the old sayin' goes, when yer mung yer Roman, you better do like yer Roman because them Cathlicks sticks together.

But I dunno why everybuddy worries about being bi-limgamal. We're all of us

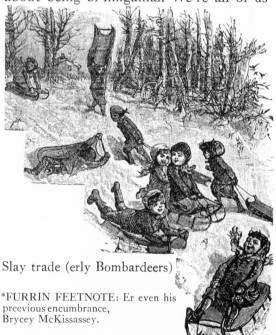

Slay trade (erly Bombardeers)

*FURRIN FEETNOTE: Er even his preevious encumbrance, Brycey McKissassey.

gonna have to lern an extra langridge in the next coupla year ennyway, and that's yer METRICAL. You won't be going to the tav fer t'order a pint; it'll be "take me to yer leeter." And you take yer tempachure. She won't be in yer Fornheit; she'll be a cent-a-grade. And the speedy limits is all gonna be changed. You won't be sluffin' thru town at 30 mile a nower; you'll be whizzin' thru at fifty kill-yer-meteors.

Now she won't be faster atall. It's all in yer mind . . . and I think that's why yer guvmint is doin' it . . . fer to make us think we're gittin' more fer our money fer to offset the inflammation. Mind you, it won't be no change fer them shrivelled servants in yer Postal Orifice to messure everything in sentipeeds. They bin movin' at yer snale's pace fer yeers.

The wife she can talk that METRICAL rite now because, bein' musickal, she's bin using yer Metric-nome fer to make time fer yeers. But myself I'm jist gonna have to git rid of that yardstick that I bin carryin' round as a rule. Looks like we're gonna be fer quite some time bi-sexed by two sets of figgers . . . even 'tho yer Yanks is gonna stick to their old standerds, which is a shame. But that's jist so much water over yer gate.

I don't think it hurts anybody to lern somethin' noo. You kin teech a real dog to take new tricks, even if she's old. Them fellas in the Postal Orifice last year went on strike over yer Otto-mayshun. They was afraid some Compewker wud come in and take away ther jobs of sittin' and sortin' and standin' and handin'. Meself, I thot yer avrage Compewker wud do them fellas a lot of good, becuz I thot a Compewker was a fella who lived in the country but worked in the city. Turns out to be a big machine that's s'posed to be inflailible like yer Pope.*

Now I can't speek fer yer Pope, but them machines can compuke up a mistake.

And when they do it's a ring-tailed snorter. I mind the time my prescription run out on yer *Plowboy* magazine.** Well sir, every month old Hew sent me a letter remainding me to join on agin at a new low price, and I never done nothin about it . . . them remainders kept comin' reglar as crockwork. Well by golly, one day they come in bags beside the road, and the old box was stuffed like a chicken at thrashin' time. I bleeve they sent me 35 thousand letters that one day fer to re-sign up to yer Gurley-Gurley mazzagine. I tell you I sent the munny in the next day. I told Heffer, "If youse want me that bad, youse can have me I s'pose." Wern't two months later I found out that Amurrikan compuker had broke down tryin' to spell the name Farquharson.***

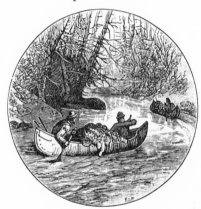

Montreal voyeurs on the rapids transit

I belong to yer United Farmers of Ontario and we bin havin' a lotta trubble with Yer Majesty's males becuz of our nishuls U.F.O. Everybuddy thinks we're them unindemnifiable flying objecks. So last year we changed ourselves to O.F.U., and now they won't even deliver our letters because they say that kinda langridge is only fit fer the Common House. (I wonder what kinda problems yer French onionist gits into with his C.N.T.U.?)

*HOLEY FEETNOTE: But yer compewker is still nondy-nominayshunal. While you take yer avrage Pope, he'd be Roamin Cathlick.

**BARE FEETNOTE: That'd be the one got out by Hew Heffer runs the Bunny Clubs fer yer *Breeder's Diegist*, and puts the stables in the girl's navals when they're center spread.

***FANETIC FEETNOTE: Dunno why. She's pernouced the way she spells it out . . . Far . . kew—har . . sin. But that's why I got all the remainders fer the hole continence.

They sure got the wind up last yeer when two unions in labor scabotaged yer Shames Bay and put the hole thing up to the Cree without a paddle. If them Injians had done the same thing, they'd all bin thrown in the whosegow without preservations. Wich makes me think that the hole ruckus was got up by yer Booracick fer to pervide extra work and live up to the tightle of that book he wrote "A Hundred Thousand New Positions," wich had got him 'lected because everybody thot it was about sex and exercised their french fries for him.

I think it's a darn shame not lettin' yer Cu-beck Injian live offa the land like his nobel incesters. Them peeples can last the yeer round on an Elk er a Moose er the odd Rotarian who needs gide-ance. But Booracic wants to flood them right up ther Straits of Um-gawa. He never waited to see if the hole thing was feasy-able. Jist bulled ahead over yer happy hunted grounds jist to prove to the rest of them Cue-beckers that he gives a dam and wants to give power to the peeple. But sounds to me it's to give more power to them peeple down on Wall Street that's alweez grabbin' at our assets.

Mind you, yer Injian fit back and got a subjunctive from yer Cort, but was over-rule the next week by a local maggotstrait. Corse, if yer Redman ever gits his land clames fer to stand up in cort, it's us that'll end up on yer reservations.

I think the things Cuebeckers do best is Expose. And I mean both yer Jarry ballers in the Park, as well as the big fare got up by that French mare Jean Drapout. Next year, he's gittin' reddy fer to show his Lymphics, and the name will probly git changed from Man on His Tare. (If he has to take money from yer Cosy Nostril fellers, it'll probly be called Man and His Underworld.) But he may jist call it Yer World Serious Expose if this ball team knocks the pennance offa yer Pissburger Pie-rats. If Cue-beckers put as much push into ther pollyticks as they done in ther orgy-nized sports, they'd take over our Common House in no time.*

I dunno how they feels about ther foot-brawlers, yer All-wets, but do you mind the time them Hocky Hibitants was in yer Stanley Cups at the Quorum and some raffyree give Rocky Richard a misconducted peenalty? My hinkus, but they had a reglar knock 'em up an drag 'em down full scales Ryet Act. Now us Ontaryans, we're the nopposit. I mind when they was makin' a hocky movie couple yeers ago and they was shootin' round our Hockey Urena and they couldn't think of what to call the name of the pitcher yet. But, well sir, the Prime Minster let slip a pare of words in the Common House by mistake, and them two words he whispered become the name of that filum: "FACE OFF."

*INDOOR FEETNOTE: Mind you, they got quite a feat in the door so far with Jean Marshland puttin' us all into Transports of Delite. And Marg Lalonde makin' his politickal footballs to prove that Lalonde is Strong.

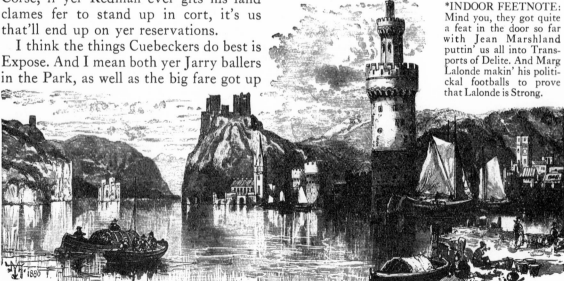

Low tide Gaspy

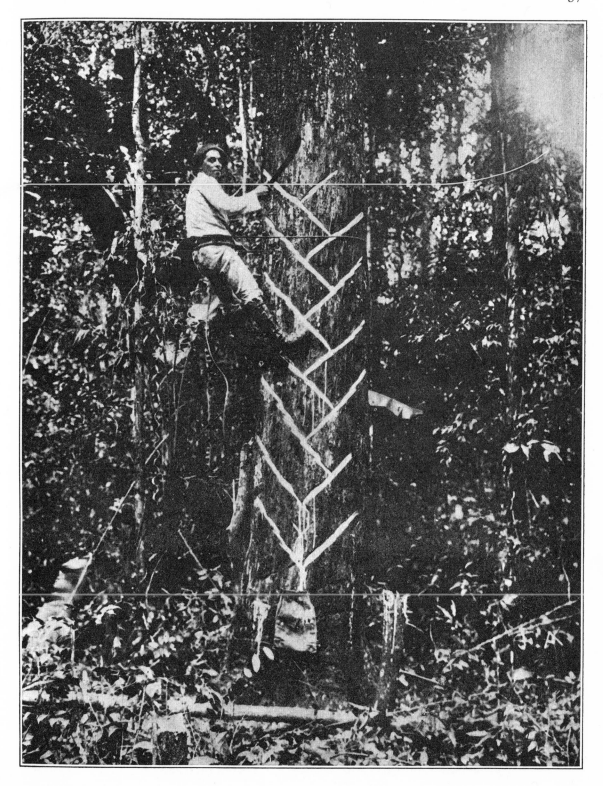

Cuebec pollen booth—seecret ballot

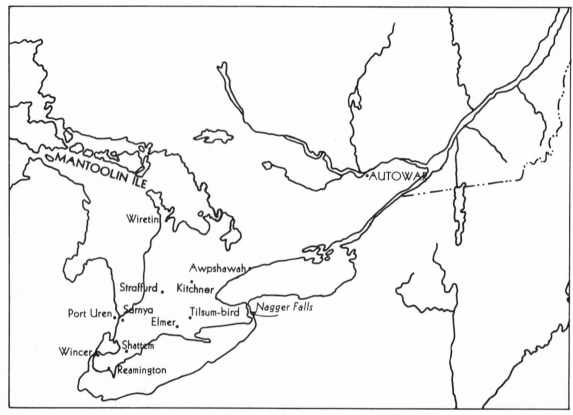

South Ontaryo

SUTHERN ONTARYO: A PLACE YOU KIN STAND?

It's best known in my famly fer bein' the gateway to Norther Ontaryo. Ontaryo is a Nindian fraze meening "rocks off in the water," refurring to the time when there wuz a lack of bars, manely sand. Tronto wuz an old Indian who helped yer Lone Rangy, and it meens "Meat-in-Place," probly becuz of the sockyards put up by some Swift Canadyans. (One thing I'll say fur them Canda Packerds, they alweez let you know wich way the wind blows.)

Offishul Flour: Yer Trillyun, in honer of inflation.

High Point: I thot it was yer Royls Winter Fare, but it's now yer CM Tely-ex-communicated Tower, that big ugly lookin' dingus denominating yer waterfront, lookin' by day like yer Iffy Tower with a mud pack and at nite like a long lit-up zipper. Yer s'posed to be able t'eat mosta the way up it on a restrunt that resolves on its axes. I'm sure not gonna take the wife up there and have to throw over a $1.75 lunch.

Sitties: That's what them sutherners got most of . . . sprawls on ther urbs.

Wincer: Acrost yer river from Deep Troit, and the only sitty we got that's in yer Deep South. Peeple here don't know wether they're comin' er goin' they got so many computers going back and fourth on yer Embarrasador Bridge. Last Janyouary, we was on our own Standerds Time, and acrost the boarder they was on ther Daylites. So it wuz offul tuff if you was a Wincer-liver and had to cross over in the dark to work . . . unless of corse you wuz a imported mugger.

Wincer makes cars, beer, wiskey, chimmicals, and all kinds of drugs. So now you know wher to go on yer next "Smiles fer Millyuns" . . . good old Hirem Walker-vill!

Sarnya: Acrost from Porch Uren. Used to be called "The Rabbits," but groath has slowed down a bit since. Big influcks during Whirld War II when they started up yer rubber plant and hired plenty of yer Pollymer crackers. Yer Sarnya mite be the terminall of yer Mackenzy's Basin pipeline if she goes thru yer States. (I'm not too thrilled meself about my soft undybelly bein' held by somebody else. I think we should be self-deficient when it comes to bein' in heat this winter.) Your U/S roote may be eezier in yer short runs, but I think it'd be safer to stick the hole rang-dang-do rite up yer Canadyan's sheeld. Otherwise, all that them farmers down by Hisspeller and Dumbo will be gittin' is a second crop of seepage.

London: On yer Tems, jist like the old one with its britches falling down. If you ast me, London Lifers is sittin' pretty with the best-lookin' lo-cal in yer providence. This place is actuary yer senter of yer twenty-pay-life bizness. Wich sounds like Kingston, but in London you don't git time off fer good behaveyer. Instead they clips yer preenyums off yer fer not takin' time out.

The sitty is fulla Middle-sexers who don't know wich way to turn, but they seem to have a good time. It was gonna be yer fuchure capital of Uppity Canda back in 1792, but Tronter grabbed ther seat.

Woodstock*: Is where yer Tems runs into yer Seeder Creak. A nice town that makes scool busses fer a living, wich is a good bizness to be in becuz them things must self-destruct from inside purty offen.

Brantfurd: Had a big cerrebration last yeer in honer of ther hunderd yeer old man Alexandy Grame Bellville, inventer of the Teflon. Them Bell mothers cellybrated by razing the rates, and the rest of us razed the roof.

Nagger Falls: Furst made famuss by Blondie doin' her tights-rope walk over a

*TOASTY FEETNOTE: Not a bad thing to have in another fool shortage.

barl. Favrit spot fer dare-devils (and even those who are too scared to git married, but only seem to register feer at yer front desk).

Berry: On Lake Simpco, at the hed of yer Campyfelt Bay, is rabbitly growing into yer Metra-popolitan Senter fer Tranna peeple who have Auto-erocketsism (crazy about driving 50 mile twice a day). Berry has awreddy incorpse-ulated the town of Alum-dale and is now spredding its testicles to include Painsick, and Shanty Bay where yer outside Plummers live.

Rillyuh: Home of grate men like Stephen LeCoq and Gord Lightfinger and a favrit of the wife's. The wife she wants to go south this winter, and we hope to git as far as Rillyuh where we has relations. And, bleeve me, yer Lake Cooch-itching is not too bad a place to have relations, s'long as you stay inside.

But yer deep southa Ontaryo fer me is jist too fulla popillation. I know cuz they all come past my place in the summertime and dumps ther garbige. I once tuk retalien-eye-ation on one of them Suthern Garberaters. I tuk down his lisensed plate, looked him up at yer Queen Parking Motory Veehickles, and dumped all his same garbidge back on his front lawn, teat fur teat.

Trawntuh: The wife and the boy are always after me fer to sell up the farm and move down to yer Metra-popollitan Hawgtown into one of them Condom-minimums. To git to yer rooms you have to go up and down in one of them Excavators till you feel like a Yo-yo . . . sept when they're on strike, when you feel like even more of a Yoyo! And the rooms is so darn small every time you cross yer laigs when yer reddin' the paper you kick the wife. Them walls is so paper thin you can alweez heer yer nabor's skeptical tank. And by gol, if they happen to leeve the lite on, you can pert neer see who flushed it.

But there won't be no more high-raisers on accounta that little Crumbie mare that tuk over from Bill Dense. He gits a crick

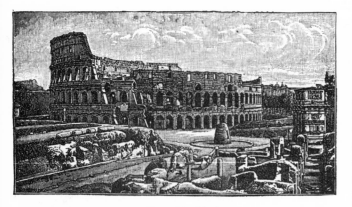

Crumbie hi-rise

in his neck from lookin' up, so he put a 45-foot limit to yer skyed-scraper. He jist told yer enveloper, "45 foot that's yer storee and yer stuck with it." Wich is why that big bilding out at Malted Airport, yer Interminable Number Two, had to git laid on its side. It was s'posed to be a uprite job, but now everybuddy has to crawl up the ellvator shaft fer to git to ther plane. It's a wonder nobuddy complaned, but I s'pose by now them sitty peeples is used to yer shaft.

One of the big problems in yer too-big sity is yer ransid transit. The subway peeple is still trying to discover yer Northwest passage, but so far they ain't made a move up yer Spadina. Someboddy's got to do somethin'. It's crowded all the time on yer McDougle and Brown Expressway,

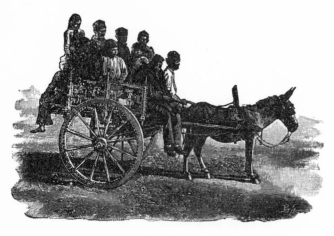

Spadina Xspressway

and they tell me that down town in yer crush hour a man is knocked down every fifteen minutes. Myself, I dunno how the poor fella stands it.

Now Billy Davis and his Queens Porkers is plannin' to have a German Money-rail, with everything above ground (goes over the heads of yer taxpayer) and without no weels touching at all fer to cut down yer syence friction. The hole rang-dang-doo has got big magnuts on the side, and its all run by hot air, jist like yer big blew machine in yer Ontaryio Legible-ature. They tried yer Go-go trains and yer Dial-a-prayer buses, and if there's one more fool shortage brung on by yer Arbs havin' us over a barl, then I think the man who's got a lotta horses to rent is gonna cleen up. (It won't stop yer pollyution. But with horses you can at least see it, and it goze good on yer peeny bushes.)

Another offal mess is yer housing. As the Anglishmen says, a man's home is his Cassel Loma, but it's gittin' tuffer'n ever to git yer wall-to-yer-wall carpet without them back-to-the-wall paymints. Even in yer sluburbs. I mind Harld Leach, one of the old Mactier Leaches (the wife she's a bit of a Leach on her mother's side), moved down to yer sluburbs of Trawntuh into one of yer split-levels in Yetobey-coke. After he moved in, he found she wasn't s'posed to be split-level. It was jist the foundation had crack, and now, by hinkus, you have to go upstairs fer to git to the seller. It's called a split-level bungle-owe, and Harld figgers it's cuz the job was a bungle and he'll owe fer it fer the rast of his days. He says when they made that house he bets they was afraid to take away the scaffolding till after they got the wallpaper well-hung.

I ast Harld wot he missed most after moving down to yer sluburbs, and he said he genrully mist the last bus home at night. He says the way sitty peeple eats out and stays out, he wonders why they have a housing crises when they could all git by with a two-car grage.

As fer yer Eldern, they don't stand a

chanct. It's eether the nursing home er the street in ther reclining yeers. Ontaryio may be a place to stand, but you gotta have a place to lie down, too. But there's so many regully-eye-ations. (We was thinking of turning our spare room into a place fer some octarino-generian, and we had a nice soft bed, roomy enuff to thrash about in. But she was only two and a half foot from the wall, and yer OHIPPY sez she's gotta be the full three feet. I think the place you'd need the three feet is in the bed, not beside it, fer peat sake. You'd think them Queen's Parker Tories would have a better understanding of yer bed-riddence when they therselves haven't bin out in thirty years.) I think they should give more of yer money fer the hostable-ization of yer old peeple, what they call yer Gerry-care, sints they gits sick more'n yer yung peeple with ther Pubicare.

Parking is a thing we don't worry about to home in our drivin' shed. But in Trawntuh, they hold youse up fer transom and are even passing laws agin it when you comes to town fer to sell yer aigs to Bloblaws. They won't even let you park at this new Zoo they got hard by Pickring, wher they plan to scare the animals with all them Dumbo jets breaking thru the wind barryer at yer new areport. Seems

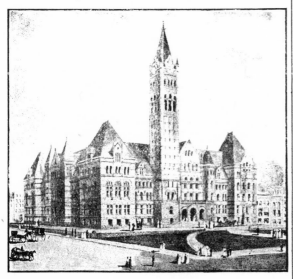

Yer farmer city hall

you have to take yer rabbits transit out ther and then walk a mile fer a camel. I s'pose that's okay fer Trawntuh peeple,

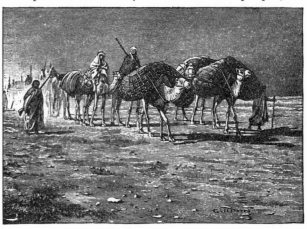

Tronto Zoo (walking a mile fer a camel)

but us outlanders has to drive all the way into yer hub with our second-hand pick-up adding to yer traffick indigestion, park it wile they rent us the space, and then spend more money fer to git on yer slub-ways fer to git out to see the Reino-sasserass and the Hippy-optimus.

Now th'oppsit sityation seems to be happenin' at yer prisns. With all them fellas excapin' into ther git-away cars parked beside them walls, it seems to be kinda Open House. Now I think we should take that fella in charge of prisms, yer Solicitus Genral Warren Almond (sounds like some kinda nut) and put him in charge of yer new Zoo. That way, we wun't have to go visit the wild animals, fer Allmand he'd let them loose every week-end and they cood come visit us in our homes.

Mind you, ther's lotsa nice places to visit down South, 'sides Trawntuh. You take **Humlton,** owner of yer whirld's flattest mountin, yer Nagger Escrapmint, and Canda's two biggest steel cumpnees, yer Smelco and yer Stinko. Mebbe that's why, when they had the garbage strike last summer, it was nine weeks before any-buddy cot on. When we was there, we dun Durn Cassle, yer Buyalogickal Garden,

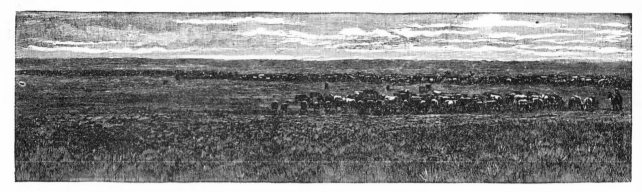

Humltun Mountin

and the Toom of yer un-noan football playr.

Gwelf is wher they have yer Agger-cultural College and give Seeminars on yer Artfishul Incrimination.*

Galt used to be nice till they called it Camebritch and fludded it out this spring. They evaccinated all the kids by helluva-copter, and you never seen so many kids in yer life. Turns out they was the same little tads oarin' back to ther homes fer to git another helluvacopter ride. We have relations there, too. The wife's second cussin twice removed . . . well, three times if you count the fludd . . . she made her way out the front door on the dinin' room table wile her husban accompaninnied her on the pie-anna.

Straffurd, hard by Shakespeer, is still Festering every yeer, tho' why they call it yer Shakespeer Festerer when they pitch

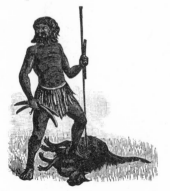

Stratfurd Festival   (actor right, critick left)

ther tent six mile down the road in Straffurd is more'n I can see. They don't have the tent no more since she got blew down by that torpeedo from Sarnya, and the guvmint made them put up the proper outbildins. But she still puts me in mind of a tent.

It's nice to sit by that arty-why-fishul lake, eat yer peeny butter sangridges, and feed the wax paper to the swans. Ya'd wunder ware they git the drane-age fer to keep the fake lake from gittin' ransid, but I s'pose they keep them swan around fer to act as a Garburator. We never had a swan for Chrissmus, but I'm thinkin' there's sich a lotta meat on that neck, she mite be better'n a goose. Mind you, she's an ugly bird, yer swan . . . peck off yer laig as quick as look at yuh, but I figger ther handy to have about fer garbidge.

We din't care fer it so much inside the tent after the Boy Scouts blew ther bugles fer the show. The play wern't by yer Beard of Avon Calling at all, but some Frenchy called Molly-Air. It was all about a fella who thot he was sick but wasn't . . . sounded to me like a lotta poppy gander by yer Christian Scientificks. I wish't we'd of gone the next nite fer to see them put on the old time clothes and git up on the platform and recite "Love's Lost When Yer in Labor." The wife she wishes we'd gone insted down to the Nagger-on-the-Lake St. Bernard Pshaw* Festerall.

*FAKE FEETNOTE: Our cattle won't take the bottle stuff 'long as they can still git draft.

*SOFT FEETNOTE: In yer Pshaw, the "p" is silent, like in swimming.

'Sides, we din't want to have nuthin' to do with that Eery Lake, wher the water is gittin' as murkry as yer fish. So we come home by way of Port Dafloozy and staid overnite at yer Landmark Muttel hard by **Sin Kathurns,** wich is the place where yer O.P.P.s streaked down 115 yung peeple fer to git at six ounce of yer Marry-jewahyena. (That's what they call that Mexican laffin' terbacco.) The papers said the yung folk was stripped, but that's got to be yer hyperthetical erra because I strip fourteen Holstein twice a day and it don't involve taking off nothin' but yer milk tubes after they bin properly hosed. I'm not too sure what reely happin't when they was serched, but it sounded like some was sent over to yer Rectall drugstore, while the rast was gone over all the way to Ragina.

I mind the time when I was down to Trawntuh near yer Yorickville and a couple of them hippos with the beerds down to ther belly-bottom drawrs arst me to step into ther pad. I told them that's the kind of thing we try to avoid in the barnyard. Turns out all they wanted was fer me to sine ther partition fer to legallyize maryjawanta, hishash, and LCD. I tole them I'd sine it if the stuff was give away free by yer MCBO but oney to peeples over the age of sixty five. I told them young tads that they cud stick an Assburn in ther Pepsy-cola, but it's yer old folkers needs the psycho-delicatessen wavy lines so's they kin have a giggle on ther way to yer last hedstoned. Why I knoo old age punshners that'd never bin on a trip as far's Nagger Falls. Well sir, they din't want me to sine it, them young hipsies. They jist waved me good-bye with what Winsome Churc'ill used to give as his V fer Victry (two figers up). I give them haff of it back.

Mebbe that's why I don't want to move down to yer south of Ontaryio. Have my boy Orville spend all nite in one of them disconnects dancing to yer Rotten Roll? I wun't mind if they all shook a boot and had a good time, but they don't seem to

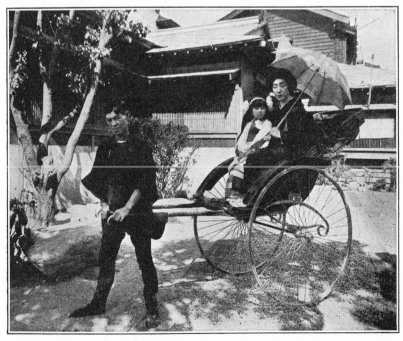

Beetin' Tronto's transit strike

move much but ther abominable mussles. Jist scrape ther feet on the floor like they stepted on sumthing. They don't hold each other, talk to each other, even look at each other. You'd think them kids had bin married to each other fer 35 year.

Mind you, Orville he's still enuff of a kid to have the best time of all with yer Canadyan Nashnul Exhibitionists. Last

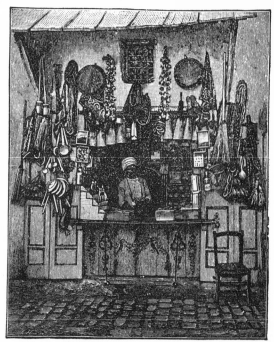

Yung Street mauler

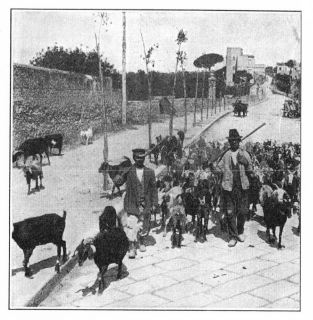

Kids' Day at C.N.E.

year they had a practickle demonstration of yer Animal Husbundry by showin' how a caff gits born. There was a couple letters in yer *Gropin' Male* from sitty peeple sayin' they din't think that sorta thing was natcheral. Myself, I think it's better'n starin' at some pore freek on yer Middleway . . . JoJo yer Dogface, walks, talks, crawls on his belly like a riptile. I think the guvmint shood give them poor unforchnates a fat LIP grant 'stedda them Yonge Street Maullers whose only projeck is asking fer yer spare change.

The wife she don't care fer yer Exhibitionists no more since she went over to yer Ontaryio Place that stands on its piles in the water. She wun't go across them piles to yer Swinesfear, becuz she can't stand hites . . . gits dizzy even when she wares

arch sports. But, by gol, she spent all afternoon at that Children's Pillage, bouncin' up and down. Said she hadn't had so darn much fun on a matress in 25 year.

Th'only thing I din't like was not finding a rest room. They got some doors with pitchers on it fer the symble-minded, but none of 'em sez MEN and LADEES no more . . . and my gol the way wimmen wear slacks nowadays, I din't know wich pitcher to go in under. Seems to me Untarryio Place is a place to stand all right, but there's no place to go. And what with yer Daylite savings, it takes an offal long time fer to git dark on them grounds.

But I'd gess Robard's big ball in the water is overshaddered by yer world's biggest rection, yer CN Telyercommunicants Tower. They say that you can sit in a restrunt at the top of that prong, look thru a pare of bye-knackerleers, and see peeple eeting offa the Needle in Nagger Falls.

Only thing the rast of yer province has got to compeat with that wud be a peek behind the curtains at yer 24 Sus-Sex Drive. If you was to ast me wot wuz the most specktackler accomplishment in the past few yeers, I'd say it was havin' two consexutive babees born on Chrissmus days. I dunno if he's gonna try fer the hat trick, but even if he rasts on his lorils he's still doin' good yer Premiere Trousseau.* The second time they was preaired fur it, and had the shepperds reddy on the Common House lawn, but the only Star in the Eest they seen was Bobby Stansfeeld. The wife and I sent the young lad a present . . . a pound of frankenfurters on accounta we din't have no gold er merr. Jist wish the Father cud run the hole country like he plans his family.

I mind the time all us farmers brung our tractors and went p'rading with our plackerds in front of yer Common House, and we wuz told to move on by yer Mounted cuz we was crematin' an offal dissembly. So we went on up to 24 Sustsex Drive and left them a note sayin', "We want more fer our milk!" We got a note back sayin' "Jist leave two quart and a pint of creem. And Chargex it."

But I'm beginnin to digest from yer Jogfree. Now **Ottawa** is not the same as **Oshawa**, 'tho both of them manage to give us the gears. But the one up yer Riddly-o Canal is s'posed to be the senter fer yer nation's capitall, altho' I bleeve they keep it perminintly down on Bay Street. The French word fer Ottawa is spelt more like "Aoutaways," wich sounds like "Way out," wich is wot everybuddy complaned at the time it was chose. Still, it's a purty histerical sitty at any time, startin' with yer statyou of Shamplane with his sextant in his hand at No-Peein Point. They gotta lotta quaint old wartime housing still standing frum Whirld War II, and I s'pose they jist can't be botherd puttin' the East Blocks to them. Yer Nashnul Wore Musemen has got almost as menny fossils as yer Sennet. Yer Nashnul Galleys has got all them paints-by-numbers of yer Grope of Seven, Tom Tomson, Jack Jackson, Jon Jonson, Jim Jimson and so on. And if you stand in front of yer Infernal flame** belching on yer front lawn of the Common House, you can hear the Carry-on swinging up in yer tower of Peacer.

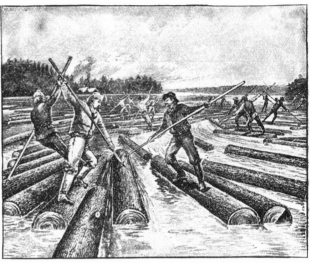

Jam sessyun in Ottawa

Ther's a lotta urbane developmint goin' up all round yer Sibillant Servant parts of town, till it's startin' to look like the old London during yer Berlitz after them German Junkies and Messysmutts got thru. Meself, I preefur **Kingston** with its quietly digglyfied limeystone bildings like yer R.M.C. and yer Pen, and yer Universality fer yer Queens. Nice thing is they all plays with eech other, speshully yer amater soft ballers from yer Miltry and yer Peenaltensionry fer to see wich is mitier, yer Pen or yer Sord. Pers'nally, I don't think yer Miltry fellas has ever got over yer Younickfication of yer Armed Forces, wich made them all wear the one uniform. That's not vurry san'tary, 'speshully in summer.

Peetie-boro on yer Trench River is a nice town, paddlin' ther own canoes.***

*P.E.T. FEETNOTE: That's French fer first wedding dress.

**HOT FEETNOTE: I coodn't find wat kinda fool they use, but it's eether sakerd or propane.

***BILINGAMAL FEETNOTE: That'd be PAS DE LEUR RHONE QUE NOUS.

And they got a nice Universty at yer Trench mouth, even tho' it looks like the movie-set fer Came-a-lot.

Cornhall and **Blockvill** is two towns that woodn't move fer yer St. Laurent Seeway, unlik yer pore Morse-burgers, and I think they was rite . . . the whole thing has turn out to be a big flop now that they're turnin all yer big otion liners into Florider huttels. Yer tooriests wants to fly now-daze, even if it meens takin' a chants on gittin' jacked off to Cuber. You mind that plain from Dubblin that was force-landed at Maltin' when yer F.I.B.s under Eefy Simbolist shot out the tires, and then she ended up in Habana? Well sir, that werked out so good, they got the reglar service from Irelind now, yer Cuba-lingus.

Thur's uther places along Lake Eery, if you kin stand them. You kin purt neer stand on Lake Eery on accounta Nixon doing his dishonerrable withdrawl of his funds fer p'lution.* Funny thing about yer p'luters, the Guvmint makes so much fuss about us gittin' the lead out of our tee-kettles when they shood be after them big fynanshul typhoons to git the lead outa ther plants.

I hear they done a darn good job of cleenin' up yer Deep Troit River from all that sympthetic oil from **Sarnya**. Mind you, yer Amurricans don't seem to do ther share, wich is why acrost the river is called Port Urin. Seems a darn shame, too, when peeple can't go into that lake fer the weekend and have a Grand Bender. I think I'd rather see yer Gorge rise along yer Nagger froot belt wher yer Canadyan Whiners lives. Even yer Amurricans is startin' to drink our ferment.**

There's good eets too, 'speshully at yer Walloper Hotel in **Kitchner** during yer

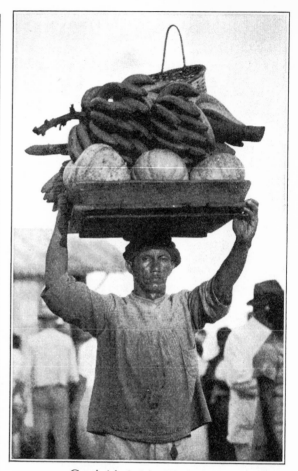

Gettin' loded in Kitchner

Oksoberfester. They throw one a the best spreds on yer road. Yer Hollander marsh gives good hed lettus mosta the times, pluss yer termaters and collieflours down **Lemmington** way. And it's worth takin' a deet-hoor up to **Ingysol** jist fer to cut the cheese. I 'spose I shu'd be talkin' 'bout yer Otto Pack towns, **Oshawa** and **Oakvill**, with yer General Mottors holding the Ford till the return of your Stewd Baker. Yer refined nickels comes from the metal urges at **Port Coalburn** on yer Well-in Canal. If yer likes big spread-out sluburbs, ther's **Misty-soggy** wat's all in the **Bramily**. But I'm gittin' homesick. To me, Suthern Ontaryo is jist yer gaitway to Parry Sound. I gess I haven't felt the same about goin' down to Trawntuh ever since last winter, when them Rosedale Gettoers put up the barrycades fer to keep out yer

*ODD FEETNOTE: I dunno why that Nixon wanted to be President of yer Eew Ass when he's alreddy leeder of yer Libbral party in Ontaryo. Funny thing, a man trying to get unpeached and impaired in two countries.

**WHINE FEETNOTE: Yer vice-president-that-was and now attorney-at-large, Spurious Agness, is s'posed to have said after swallering some, "I'd rather be Bright's than President."

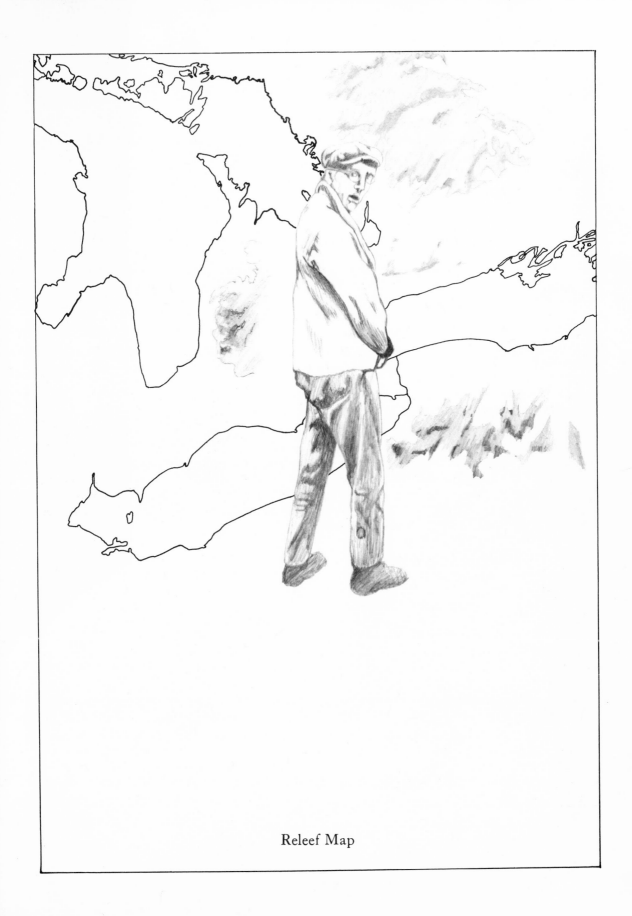

Releef Map

middlin' class. Made me feel like a reglar Checked-point Charlie.

Anuther thing about Trontuh bothers me is yer Yung Street Since-strip with all that adulterated fornoggrefee in yer moovy houses, speshully in the summertime when they has yer Maul. Now I know sum peeple likes bean accostered by yer Alkyholicks Unanimuss, and yer Hairy Krishnuts with the pidgin paint on ther fourheds. But meself I like to keep to meself without bean told to go into a belly-rub parler and git rubbed the rong way by some topfull mass-use. I dunno why them Maulers is so poplar (yew musta herd that song "Bless the Maul"). I think it's the falt of that Dr. Spock (the peedy-asstrushun with the funny eers used to be on yer Star Dreck with thut fella who's now Captin in charge of yer Bob Loblaws, Willyum Shatnurd). He's the fella sed you shoodn't spank yer kids . . . and now that they've groan up, ther jist dyin' to have

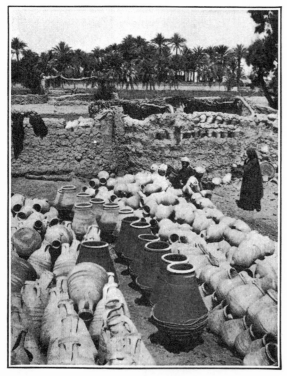

Aftermass of pot raid
on motel (a Land Mark)

some stranger hit them on their south forty a few times fer to eeze their gilt edges.

But it's yer moovie that gits me the most. You try to find a unadulterate fillum fer to take a fifteen yeer old to, down among Tronto's tendererloins. It's eether "Kung Fu You Too" or "Gang Bang Yer Dead." And when you do find one you wanta see, they won't let the boy in cuz he ain't had his majority like Primestir Trousseau. That's how we missed out on "Lassie Go Homo" and ended up bringing up yer tail of a long line at yer "Exorsass-assist." I dunno how it's pernounced. I thot it was mebbe a fella doin' push-ups, but Valeda sed it was one of them Bible pictures like the one with Peter Toole (funny how he repeets hisself like that), when he plaid God hisself, on camera as well. I liked the book better. And I mind I dint care too much about that Pope film, "Cardinal Knowledge." But annyways, we went in to "Yer Exercisist" becuz Valeda sed it was about the Devil gittin' busted fer possession.

Well, sir, if you thot there was a long line outside yer theeyater, yu shooda seen the one inside fer the warshroom. And no wunder. I was kinda sorry we missed our dinner standin' in line, but if we'da had it we'da missed it anyways. It's the one pitcher I wished parts of wasn't in yer Tecknickle-culler. The wife and boy spent mosta yer moovy under the seet, and with people rushin' by them to yer W.C.'s and yer M.C.'s too. There was consuderable laying on of hands by feet. Finely, Orville he hadda git up and go to the rast-room, but when he got there the line-up was still so long that he coodn't wait. Then he seen that little box the Salivation Army has on the wall wich sez "Fer the Sick," so he used that. I'm sure glad they brung back that pitcher with Mary Poppins jumpin' offa yer Alp in "Yer Sound of Mucus."

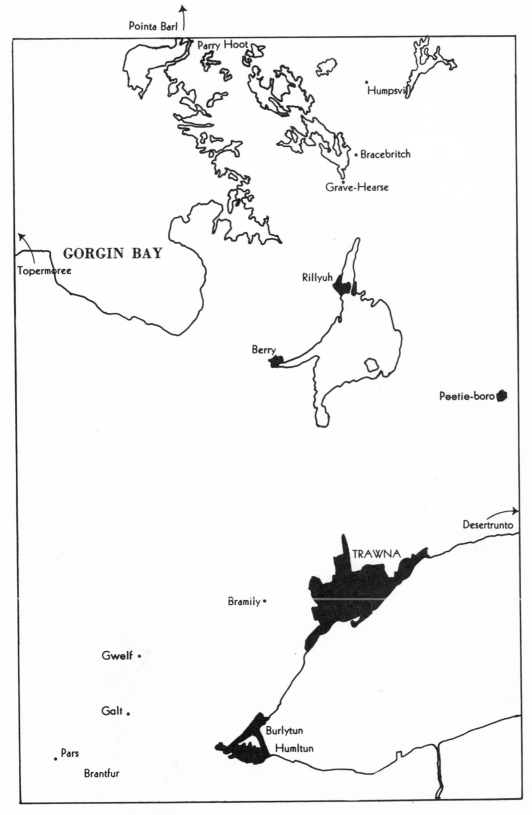

Parry Hoot and Envy-irons

NORTHREN ONTARYO

It's nice to git back home and away from all that garbidge down south, sept that yer Trontonarians is starting to deport ther refusals up our way. 'Stedda decomposting it therselfs, they're gonna have a dump on us. I think it's caused by yer Queens Porkers with ther infernal regional guvmint, tryin to turn good arble land into what they call yer green belts fer yer wreck-creation.* And one of ther plans for us Northners is to send us all ther Effluent.

Now I allus thot yer Effluent was yer rich peeple . . . turns out to be a fancy word fer the crap throne out by yer rich peeple. And they're gonna pile it all up our way till it gits to be a mountin, and then when it gits cold enuff so's you don't mind the smell, they're all gonna drive up here and ski on it. You think I'm kiddin'? It's called yer Mable Mountin, and it's expecktorate high among yer wintered reesorts. But I don't think sitty peeple is gonna drive over four hundrerd mile jist to have some ups and downs on ther weakend. They should take all them plastical bags and make a Green Belt outa yer Humpilton Mountin. That could do with sum elevatin'! She's not much more than a plat-o. Then yer Rosedalers and yer Forestry Hillers from Tranna cud drive only forty miles fer to slide on ther slats.**

Us Northmen got enuff trubbles without goin' downhill some more. Come the cold wether and she's slipry out, the wife sure wud like to have a cuppla studs under her, but yer pervincial guvmint don't allow it. Insted, they want us to buckle up our casualty belts, and they're thinkin' of makin' it repulsory.

Mind you, it don't do no good 'less you got the kinda belt crosses yer hart and under yer pectorials, fer jist the belly-band kind only garntees that haff of you will

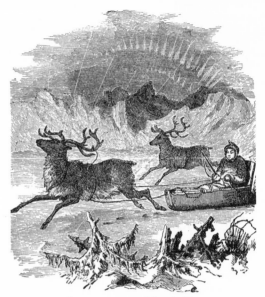

Stag party at North Bay

stay in the car. So buckle up yer overhed, fer it's better to be safe than shorty. But winter's even tuffer on pederastrians up our way. I mind when the wife tuk the dog out fer a walk, and they tell youse fer to ware white on yer hieway. By swinjer, she was all white . . . white fur hat, white raincoat, white mitts, white rubber boots, and white dog. And darned if the two of 'em didn't go along the side of the rode that nite and git run down by the snowplow.

I think a lotta sutherners that worships yer Mother's Nature all summer shud try comin' up in Febyou-ary and sit in our two-holer with nothin' on hand but a frozen corn-cob. You ast my boy Orville if it's much fun gittin' outa a warm bed at six o'clock in the mornin', and strait out onto a cold bike-sickle seet. But seams sitty peeple can't git enuff of yer Grate Outdoors. I s'pose it's only us ruriels that worships yer Grate Indoors and don't spend no more time outside then we has to. Even in summer when them musqueeters start dive-bomming us from Pointa Barl, it don't do to stay out, sints that spray they give us after they cansselled yer D.D. and T. don't do much more than give the buggers a perfumed sitzbath. They jist

*SHADY FEETNOTE: Pee-Air Terdo musta had a green belt oncet, but it turnered brown from doin' the Judy-o.

**SLIDIN' FEETNOTE: As the pote sez, if yer mountin won't go to Humltun, then Humltun'll have to go to yer mountin.

take off refresht, do a couple circuses of the feeld, and sink ther stinger agin.

But that don't stop the same strangers comin' back year after year. They're alweez stoppin' at our vegetubble stand fer to ask if the things is orgasmically groan. If you ast me, all that orgasmic stuff is jist a lotta horsemanoor. I got a pile of it thirty feet high outside my barn, and that's the stuff them sitty peeple incests on havin' on ther strawbreez. And them same peeples will bild a swimmin' pool not ten rod from a lake and surround it with that arty-why-fishul Asstero-turf like they have in yer Doomed Stadyum in Euston, Texass. When I hear that, I'm glad I live on the farm wher you can live in peese and digglity and fight with the wife without bein' herd.

Mind you, the boy, Orville, he don't want to be a Northern Ontaryan. He wants to hed south fer to finish his eddifi-cation in one of them Trade scools, yer Disco Tech. I'm hopin' he'll stay to home since the guvmint finely took the curse off yer Suppression Dutys, and Orville can de-herit the farm with'ut me havin' to pertend I'm his hired hand and give it over to him before I go into the Behind of yer Beyond. 'Corse now, they have a kerb on yer land. I thot at first that itt'd be good to have a curb, fer when yer out in the feelds it's too much trubble to go all the way back to the house. Turns out it's not that kind of a kerb. Jist the guvmint makin' it hard fer us to sell-out to some millyunair from Cleeveland.

And then we got yer Reegionals guvmint foist on us from outside. I think the Departmint of Munipissipal Affairs shud stick to ther own. Do you mind the time Trawntuh got amangle-mated up, and didn't them sluburbs kick up an offal stink not to join Hawgstown? I mind the

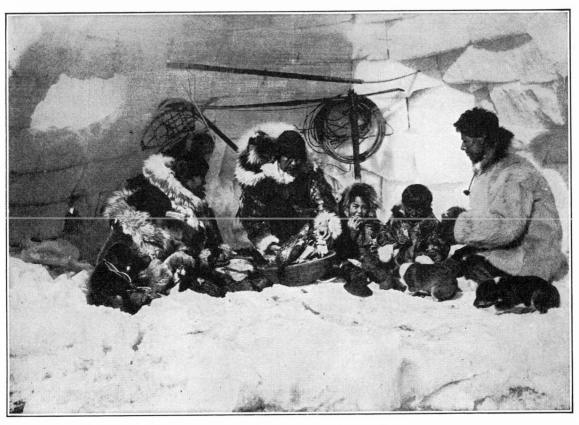

Chrismus at the cottidge — Pointa Barl

slogun they had: "Divided we stand, yewnited we fall." They was jist drug in fer to pay fer that new slubway with all them fancy bathroom-tile stashuns. Well, that's the way us R.R. #2 McKellar-dwellers feels about being incorpsulated into Megalopolitan Parry Hoot so that us outlanders is gonna have to pay fer all flushable toilets in Metropopolitan Parry Sound wile we're still stuck on our old skeptical tanks.

Not that we aren't proud of our town. Our big Boston Broozer Bobby was born jist around the corner from Main street in the old Orr house. His weddin' was the biggest thing to hit Parry Sound since the Green stamps. I haven't seen the wife so excited since she fell offa the roof. Mind you, nobuddy got to go there 'septin' mebbe yer broom's mother. He purt neer din't make it hisself, bean out on Blackstone Lake cuz yer muscle-lunge had started to bite. But I wanta creck somethin' said in the papers beneeth the bride's pitcher. It sed, "Mrs. Orr nee Peggy Wood." I want to say rite here and now that no sich thing happen'd. Bobby's mother, Miz Orr, has never bin noan to lay a hand on anybuddy, much less start out her son's married life by giving the bride one with her nee.

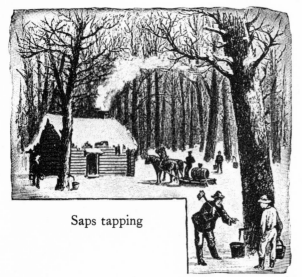

Saps tapping

Bobby he's not jist in the hockey, ya know. He has the lingery store on Main Street whur he sells maternity close fer yer Modren Miss. Wich is handy becuz jist this yeer he got a little defence-able-man of his own. (Well, ackshully the wife bored him, but Bobby got the assist.)

My gol, here I am talkin' about the home town when there's all the rest of yer vast-froze Northland, too.

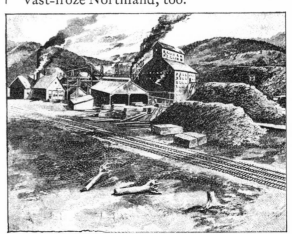

Niggling in Subbery

Now, you take **Subbery**, yer Rock capitol of Canda, even tho' it's a town divide aginst itself by yer ralerode tracks. But when it comes to minin' its own bizness, there's yer **Copper's Cliff**, yer **Fallenbritches**, and yer **Nickel Change**. And **Elliott Late**, named after Prime Minster Trousseau's marridge. The town has as its slowgun the thing that Premeer is 'sposed to have whisper'd to yer Opposite Position: "Up Yeranium!" **Norse Bay** on Lake Nopissing (not too strickly in force) is the gaitway to Parry Sound, Macteer, and Nobel (wher every yeer they give out the prizes fur peece). Norse Bay is not too far from **Calender**, where yer Quintuplicates was conceeve all at once. **Kapusskissing** is wher they make Kleen-eggs and forst fires, wich is caused by car-less smokers and stag parties in yer woods. I don't meen to sound like Smokey yer Bore, but my gol I can't begin to add up the holy-cost of last summer. I know sum

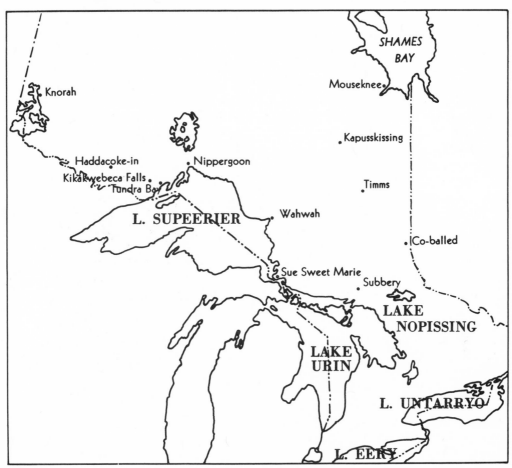

Northern Ontaryo

of it was caused by yer Syence friction from yer lightning having spontainyous indigestyun. But there's too many peeple with careless butts, and them Camp tipes thinks you can make a little heat by rubbing two Boy Scouts togither.

Up north is yer **Co-balled** and yer **Cockran.** The first is a musuleeum, and the second is still a nice bushy town. **Haleyburied** and **Newly Skeered** is up ther, too. One had a silver belt, and t'other still got its green belt (fer four munts anyways). My gol, how can I forget **Timns** now that we're back on yer Gold standerd and Bookavetchy's store will start givin' out green stamps agin to yer Muckytire minors. Over at yer Grate Divide (I meen Lakes Urn and Speerier, not yer Departmint of the Infernal Texa-

tion) we got **Sweet Saint Marie,** home of yer Phill and Tony Expose-atoe, yer well-noan scorer and your shut-out King.

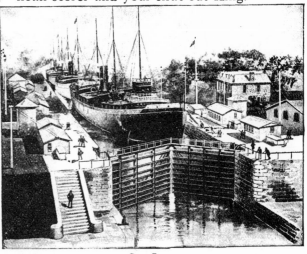

Sue Lox

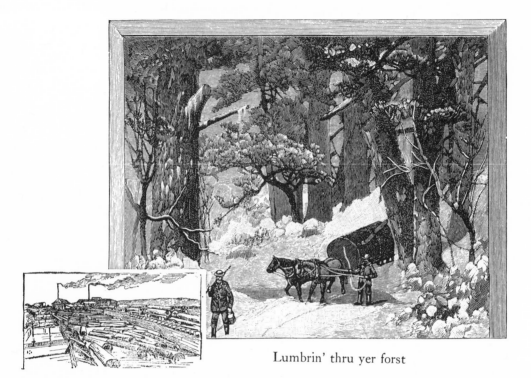

Lumbrin' thru yer forst

Makin' kleenex

But even further north, lotsa tooreeists is startin' to go all the way. (I'm not talkin' bout what goes on in yer muttels, but way up there on yer Jameses Bay hard by yer **Moosesnee.**) Yer Poler Bare train takes yez up to wher you can see the big white fuzzy things fer yerself, as well as wall-russ (yer beerdy seel) and them birds called Artick ptare-migins. (Don't ask me what a bird's doin' with a "p" in the front.)

Way, way over west on yer Lake of the Hoods is **Knorra,** wich has got more Injians than you can shake a stick at, and they git it shaken at them quite reglar. Last summer, they started shakin' it back, and got help from some of ther Amurrican brothers from Woondy Nee, 'tho I don't think they reely wanted it. But they sure need help from summers. Becuz that parkland in Knorra was took away from yer Injian in the first place. So I don't blame them fer goin' in there and pitchin' ther tense.

Last but not in yer leest, yer Lakes Heads, Pore Arthur and Far Twillyum, both of wich has now bin c'lectivized into **Tundra Bay** ('cept on Sardy nites, when yer fur still flies). The old Fert now lyes in roons, but yer Minster of Two-hoorism wants to re-obstruct it fur visiters. It's up ther hard by yer Kickaquebeca Falls. But do you think they want to do it on the same spot? Nossir. That'd be too easy. 'Sides, yer CPR is on that land and they wanna stay ther and roon it in ther own way. So yer guvmint is gonna bild a brand noo Fert fer mebbe ten millyun dollar. Brand new, mind yuh. (It'll take an offal lotta toureeists before that Fert will be a wreck like the old one was run over by yer CPR.)

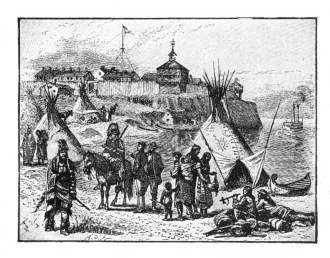

Erly Bay Daze — Dores open 9 A.M.

YER PRAYERY PROVINCES

They're called that becuz they bin brot a lotta times to ther kneez. If it wusn't rust or drout, it were grassedhopper, catterdepiller, frate rates, or yer rale strikes. This last spring, they just cum thru forty days of rain followed by yer genral 'lection (wich means sixty daze of hot air). The only remdy fur eether is to take out a big doze of Crap Insuriance.

Trubble with sitty peeples is they think that everything is dessided by eether yer capitailists on yer Sock Market er yer Shrivel servants up next yer Common House putting everything down high wide'n hansard. But when you gits down to yer bredbasket, the farmer's the one what fills it. 'Pending on yer wether, a course. The risk in yer sock market is nuthin' to sprayin' yer seed on the ground. This yeer it was so wet out West they cooden' touch the feelds till Joon. Some farmers felt so up in the air they hired airyplanes to do it fer them. (My gol, I've herd of gittin' married by correspondents, but it must take a lot of faith to spred yer seed from 2000 foot.)

MANYTOBER

It's a Chipaway word meenin' "the place where everybody comes togither to pertake of yer Grate Spirits."

The hole province is flat mosta the time, wich is mebbe why it's offen called "that floody place." It used to be all underwater and was called Lake Aggiesez, a big puddle left in the middle of us when we all got defrosted 10 thou yeer ago. Aggiesez was bigger'n all yer Grate Laiks put together, but she's gone now, and whut's left is divvyed up into Lake Winpeg and Lake Winpegoldeye-oasis. Sometimes the water it all comes back, but when it does they don't call it Lake Aggiesez agin. They just call it disastervill, and Ottawa sends water-wings to all yer dry farmers.

Clime-it: In summer, grate wether fer 'skeeters. They have a reel epedermis every year. Last summer, fer extras, they got cattypillows a foot deep. Since cutting off yer D.D. and Tease, the kinds of catterdepilatories they allow wun't even give them creepy slugs a hedache, so they go on defoley-aging.

In winter, don't ask. It's cold enuff to freeze the nuts on yer Fort Garry bridge.

Porridge La Prayry

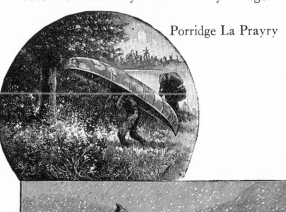

Porridge and Main

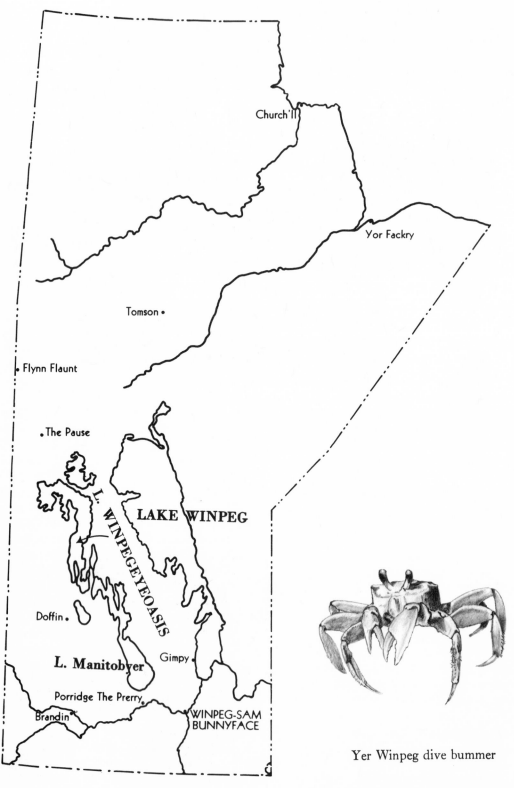

Church'll

Yor Fackry

Tomson •

• Flynn Flaunt

• The Pause

L. WINPEGEYEOASIS

LAKE WINPEG

Doffin •

L. Manitobyer

Gimpy

Porridge The Prerry •

Brandin •

WINPEG-SAM
BUNNYFACE

Manytober

Yer Winpeg dive bummer

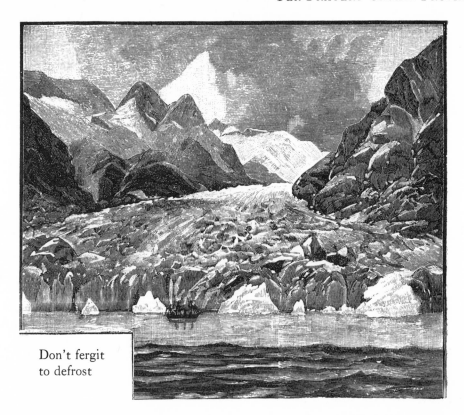

Don't fergit
to defrost

High Point: Not much: It's the top of Porkpine Hill hard by yer Boffin Lake, and I'll bet that's not as high as yer molson Golden Boy on top of yer Legible-later Bilding. Most 'Peggers think the high point is on Mane Street when the wellfare checks is give out.

Vegetatin: Lotsa weet in yer south, but up horth is forsts with mossy bottoms, wich don't hardly ever dry, so popillation is scarce. What's not moss is mustkeg, wich is nothin' to do with compulsurly drinkin', but is jist another word fer bogs (wich is where you hed fur compulsurly after drinkin').

Trees: Covers sixty purrscent of yer upper public area, mostly yer jacked pine and ballsome, not to mention yer Blacks Pruce and them white birtches. Lotsa pulping goes on at The Paw, where everyone greets ya frendly and gives ya the shakes.

Grains: Now yer talkin'! All yer Red River serials is good on accounta the valley soil is pure black Jumbo. Number One Hard Spring is yer best bet. Altho' some gits a rise out of Number Two Smutty.

Mines: Don't tell Subbery, but when it comes to making nickels, **Tom'son** has the biggest complex in the whirld. And over at **Lack Due Bonnet** (French: "Can't pay fur the hat") is yer biggest tantalum mine on yer continental. I thot this wuss used in the makin' of tantalizers fer yer mill towns, but turns out to be a bloo-gray dust fer puttin' on yer 'lectronic conductors and rubbin' ginst yer Cat-hoed toobs. (I looked that up in yer Britannicker Syclepeedriast.) The big smelters are at **Flynn Flaunt,** named after yer movie acter that swashed his buckle better'n anybody (and also had his trubbles with miners).

Yer Fish: After Ontaryo and Elberta, Manytober is the fishyest province (Number Three . . . we fry harder!) Mind you, they farm them, teeching trouts fer to seed under water. You can't teech that to a sammon; ther always goin agin yer currant. Home groans is yer Winpeg Goldyed, yer sogger (must be an extry wet fish), yer Northern piker, and yer peckrel.

River Complaint: Now Manytobans is draned by two big rivers, the Nelson and the Churchill. But the guvmint wants to change the root of these natcheral water intercourses and make them floe t'other way, retter-o-active agin Mum Nature. You take the Churchill, what floes into Hudsome Bay hard by where yer Poler bares its teeth on the garbitch dump. Well sir, yer Golden Boys in Winpeg want her to rush the other way into Injin Lake. That's where our aboriginal Canadyans makes a livin' outa fishin' and keepin' ther traps open. If there hole hauntin' grounds gits innunderdated, yer Injin won't have a lake to stand on.

Mind you, the Manytoba guvmint may change all this. It seems no matter hoo they are, Sociablelists like Ed Shry er Retrogressive Preservatives like that Walter Weerd that was, they all seem turble fond of flooding . . . and want more of it. I gess Ed Shry wants to show the voters he gives a dam, like Walter Weerd before him. But some of them ear-gation projecks has bin more ear-tation than anything elts. You take yer Gardner Dam was s'posed to make yer Prayerys blossom into yer Gardner Spot of yer Uni-worse. Well, I know farmers who thinks they was better off being hy-and-dry-landers. Fur a dam is jist a ded lake reddy fur to silt to the hilt, and all that stankant water brings on is yer Manytoba muskeeter . . . and yer western stinger is quite a breed.

I mind standing on the corner of Porridge and Main having two of them jivebomming over my head. I thot at first they was barn swallers or even chicky-hocks, but they was yer Red River muskeeters. I dunno if I was deleteerious er not, but I cudda sworn I herd one of them whine, "Shall we take this one down to the river, or eat him here?" And the t'other one whined back, "Aw, let's eat him here. If we take him down to the river, them big ones'll take him away from us!" Now you

probly think I'm ex-adge-gregatin', but it's a noan fack that yer single muskeeteer can lay 30 thou aigs a day . . . and there's no tellin' how many yer marryied one gits laid. Here's a tip fer tooriests lerned from a Manytoba natif. If a skeeter lands on yer fourhead, go ahed and slap it, but don't remove the corpus: leave it ther fer bait.

Peeple: Manytoba is a reglar Untied Nations. Besides yer French (sum of hoom are Matey) and all them Angled Saxons, everybuddy seems to have a Uke next door. And even the Icemen cometh in reglar from a place called **Gimpy**. Some Anthropoid Ollojists is fixin' to proove that yer Icelander is reely jist a Nirishman who stopped haff way fer some Ice. But my gol, I'm part Ulcer Irish and I never yet seen the one who ain't prepaired to go all the way.

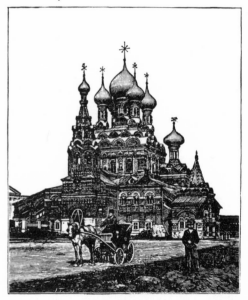

Sunday morning in Winpeg

Winipeg: Yer dead senter of yer continence,* this sitty is forth largess in Canda, 'speshully if you inclood Porridge La Prayery, Brandin, Carmen, Vergin, and Sin Bunnyface acrost the river, where yer French quarters. By the buy, Sin

*LIVE FEETNOTE: Sept on Sardy nites.

Bunnyface has nothin' to do with that *Plowboy* maggotzeen got up by Hew Heffer, so don't go brandon it as sich. The closest Sin Bunnyfacers come to that kinda life is ther weakly gambols at Our Lady of Perpetchyouall Bingo.

Winpeg is a culchural senter (besides yer horta and yer agruh, I meen). Ther mane clame to fame come from yer Royl Winpeg Footstompers, wich since it's bin foundered has probly kept yer oldest Belly dancers in Canda.

Church'll: (named after yer local custom of saying good-bye with two fingers up) is at the head of yer big bawdy of water, yer Big Bay. (Acshully, yer big head of yer Bay lives in Winpeg, but that's another storee.)

I s'pose pack ice is the main industree in the winter. That, and keepin' warm and tryna be happy. But in winter, as they isolate therselfs with spanknum moss,

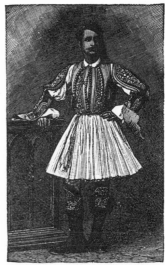

Royl Winpeg belly dancer

even yer poler bares gits down in the dumps.

Summer is the two frosty-free months when yer ice-breakers comes in to bust up

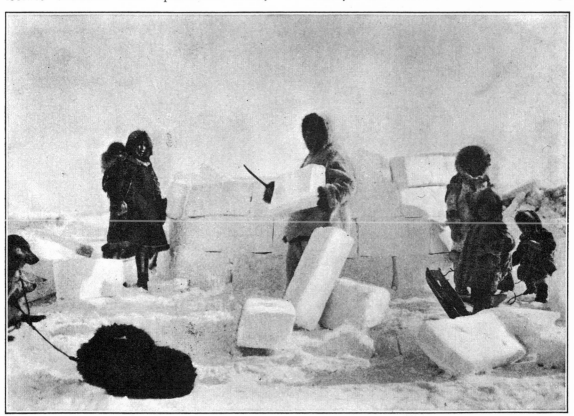

Churchill icebreaker

the pack. After yer ice-breakers, the party gits under way. S'ply boats come in twice a yeer fur to pick up males, and grane boats come in **to** yer Great White Ellvaters fer to git loaded at the same time by standing three to the brest. Fer two months Churchill-by-the-See is yer wirld's biggest grains export. The resta the time bizness is closed dew to yer ex-screams of tempachure. Other boats bring in other things, lik supplys fer yer DEWEY line (must be old Republickans who moved up here becuz they don't hold with Nixon), and other peeple willin' to try the luck of the North . . . prosspeckers, fur traiters, and yer Church peeple, becuz in winter there is lots of mishunerry positions to be filled.

Yer Future: Purty much the same as in yer pastyure. The only new industree fer Manytoba is that new Air Canda repare depot, wich come out of that promising 'lection campane last summer. (The mane thing it's s'posed to repare is Manytober's relations with Ottawa.) Mebbe it'll turn out to be anuther white ellvunt like yer 64 millyun dollar they spent fer to dig a re-moat around Winpeg. Nobuddy's figgered wether the big ditch is to help yer lo-cal dykes when they flood er jist to discurge Easterners from Knorra. I dout yer ladder. Westerners is noted fur ther hospiddleality. As the old song sez, they don't have a scourgin' werd to be herd in this land where yer dear and yer bufflo used to play, and yer Aunt eloped.

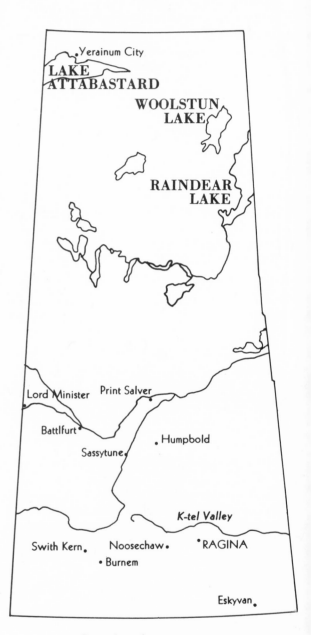

Sassakatchewon

SASQUATCHYOUWAN

It's a old Cree word wich means, "My gol, that's a swift curnt!" (I think we all suffer from this translater, and I can't tell yuh the aboriginal. But, as that pote wunce sed, "I think that I shall never see a pome luvlier than by a Cree".) Swift curnt is shure easier to spell than Sassakatchyuhwun. I feel like the Yank toorst hoo ast where he was in Canda and, when they sed, "Saskytoon, Sassakatchewon," he kep on drivin' till he got to a place wher they spoke Anglish.

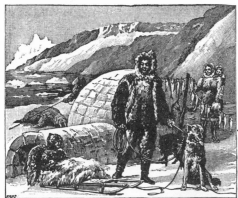

Poor Sask. farmer in winter

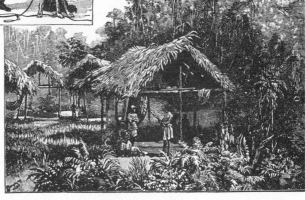

Rich Sask. farmer in winter

Yer Topplegraffy: Sask. (if you don't mind, I'll bring it up short) is what yer jografters call a peony-plane. This meens it's total flat sept fer the odd bush, or the odd rise in yer Sidepress Hills and them lasting depressyuns in yer K-Telle Valley. They even got so self-conscientious about it up Saskytoon way that they went out and bilt a mountin by hand, becuz ther winter sports got tired of bein' told to go jump in the lake (wich was also man-maid, bein' sluffed off from an old slew).

Water? And that brings me up to yer Sask. water, wich has the taste you hate twice a day. I cannot tell an alky lie. It comes from yer sluff, wich some calls slew, becuz that's what you feel like doin' to yer bellboy who brung it up in the first place. Most of this water lies in yer alklye lakes, wich is shaller basins untapped since yer Ice Age and purty well caked with slime-stone. This discourges yer groath of trees, which is mor poplar in the north but a bit of a birch in the south.

Wind: Like Bob Dillion sez, the anser is blowin' all the time.

Peeple: Hard workin', mosta them evolved in yer 4-H. (I don't meen the yung peeple's orgy-nization — Head, Hand, Hart, Hoof'nmouth. I'm talkin' bout yer Heave, Heave, Heave, and Hernya.) These peeple gits the heaves from scrapin' a livin' offa the swet on ther brow . . . and scrapes more offa ther boots before they comes in to wash up.

Producks: Mostly hard red weet, wich is groan and sold to Serviet Roosia after bar-ginning with yer Hard Reds. This all de-pends on yer Otto Pack, wich has nuthin' to do with yer Genral Motives in Oshawa. It's what sacks yer wheeter-deeler Otto Lang is able to pack on the backs of both Lioneed Brasney and Masty Tung.

It warn't too long ago when Sask. far-mirs all came a-cropper when yer weet was left in yer pools unsold. That was when yer guvmint of yer Feds step in and told them to grow the one crop and paid them to cut ther ache-rage in haff. Then yer Common House tried to set them on to rape, but some felt too old fer that. Others had so many beefs agin the guv-

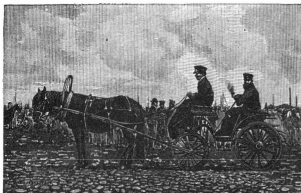

Benet buggy

Wheet car pool

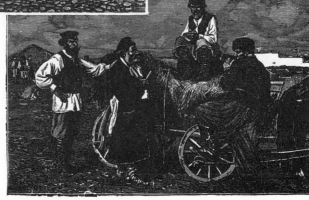

mint they even bred cattle, and still others went into hawgs. But the guvmint said "No Porking" and sudsiddy-ized them fer to stop breeding. Farmers hadda send off to Ottawa fer pamfulets to tell them what kinda feed they shud plan not to give them hawgs they was plannin' not to raze. Some of the yunger farmers jist give up and sat up haff the nite smoking pot-ash.

Some farmers neer Wayburn uncoverd oil, wich was not fur export, but good enuff fer to give yer domesticks consumption. One man who found oil on his farm sold out fore times, and eech time he did he found another farm with oil on it. Got so his frends started calling him Yer Wizard of Ooze. He's rich now, but still tryna find a peece of land to farm without no pesky oil on it.

Even 'tho they might be havin' a good time around the corner, Sassykatchers is a bit leery of posteerity, becuz they bin thru yer 1929 crash corse before. Fer a flat provinse that's not s'posed to have any ups er downs, they sure spent a long time

in the thirities in yer troff of a dip depress-yun. Mind you, they never done what them sock-brokers down on yer Walls Street done after reading ther sticker tapes—jumped offa the skyscrapes to a defnit concussion. Yer Sasky sons of toil coverd with tons of soil jist had to grit ther teeth (and them without teeth, grit ther gums) ... and ther was plenty of grit to go round. They had to wate fer somthin' constructive to happen, like World War II.*

Nowadaze there's a billyun dollars a year in grain. And mebbe this winter the hole province can git to Florider's Dizzy Wirld on ther creditible cards. But if you talk to peeple as went thru yer dirty therties drouts, they say that tho' it wuz no picanick, they mostly stuck it out without turnin' to drink—even tho' they cood reed the handwritin' on the floor. And if

*BOOT FEETNOTE: I know that shud be Wirld War Two, but them's Roamin Numerals. And there's so many Eye-talians cum over lately that yer pollytishuns is afraid to loose ther vote. How do you think Daisy Lewis got plucked?

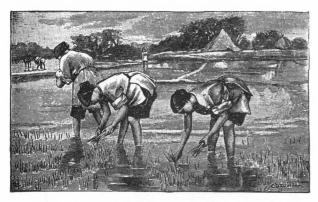

Sowing weet last spring

they got cot by the shortedges agin, I think Sassacatchewins will be better pee-paired than most, 'speshully if yer Arbs and Lesbians from yer Bayroute gits us over a barl agin. These peeple (the Sasks, I mean) will jist go back to yer one-horse-power Bennett buggy, wich don't need no gas and makes it own naturul polly-ution.

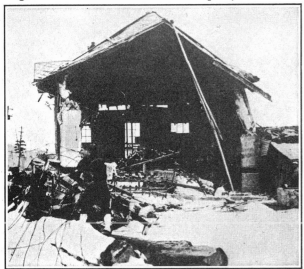

Yer dust boll after flush times was over

Before that fool crysis happint last year, yer hevvy draft horse was becumming obsoclene, jist like yer hevvy over-draft farmer. But when them oil prices goes up agin, I'll betcha there'll be a lotta sitty peeple walkin' up and down yer stalls at yer Royls Winter Fare thinkin' about turnin' in ther Cadlacks. As long as you got a horse with its own infernal combus-

tin enjun and a buggy beehind, you won't be missin' Linkun Count-nentils.

Xports: I gess the most famuss produck from here that they send out reglar wood be yer Long John Doofenbeaker, the Prints of Saint Albert. (Er is it yer Saint of Prints Albert?) Anyways, he's the grand old infanturrible of polltnicks, and a party all by hisself. He's allus bin his own man and his own Loyl Awpoosishun,* even when he was Prime Minister and brung out his own Billa Rites. Not to menshun his fame-uss Dubble Vision about opening up our hardened Articks.

I wooden be spryzed to see John cleenin' the ring round his hat and gittin' reddy fer to fillabluster at yer next leedership convenshun of yer Retrogressive Preseratives. I think he'd like to fix the party of what ales it (John thinks it's yer Dalton Cramps), before Little Jack Horner sticks his thumb in.

Saskytune: Has gotta be the helthiest sitty in Canda on accounta all the fissical jerks they got. (I'm talkin' 'bout yer Partissi-paction program of repulsory exorcises got put on them by Pee-Air Torso, who is one of yer bigger athaletic sporters.) Fer some time now they bin on a quota of set-ups, pushy-ups, and joggin' off around the blocks.

My gol, I don't think I could touch my knees without bending the floor but I know an old fella out in Saskytune, 72 yeer old, kin wrap his legs around his neck like a reglar extortionist. Every mornin' he stands on his hed fer to let the blood rush past his eyebrows, then does all them callousthinicks, has a ice cold shower and a hard rub-down with a stiff brush, and then he tells me he feels Rosy all over.

And jist think, the hole town is Sasky-tuned up like that. No wunder they bilt a mountin by hand.

Ragina: Yer plain sitty of yer Queens (Ragina means Queen, ya no) is on Lake Washcanner (fore fut deep) and is located

*BOUND FEETNOTE: Most peeples thinks of ther wife as the Loyl Opposite-posishun, but John he says that life to him is one long Marteeny . . . s'long as there's an Olive in it.

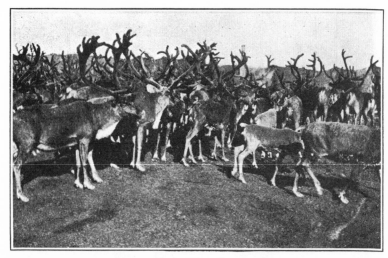

Prints Albert Elks Convenshun

entirely on the rong side of the tracks. It's yer capitalist sitty, now that weet is back on yer Hits Prade and yer Stook market is up agin. Only problem now is a shortedge of farm equipment, wich stops the combines goin' aginst the grain. The John Deere warehouse here has bin sending out lotsa "Deer John" letters to unrequited farmers.

Culcherly, Ragina is famuss fer havin' the world's shortest statyew, wich is deddicated (but not too much) to Louis Real in honer of Canada's first Sibil War. Not only did yer guvmint cover the expanse, but also a part of Louie after yer local art crickets had a full frontle look and deesided he shood git draped. Ragina is also the home quarters of the fellas what got Louie well-hung, yer R.C.M.P., noan all over the whirld as yer Musickal Writers with the cherry cotes and the Boyscout hats.

Yer Mounted is the best pleece force in the wirld, accorn to yer Sovern, Queen Lizabeth, way back yeer before last when Her Imperious Majesty come to their tencenty-all celibations. And the best pleece forces incloods Scotchland Yards with ther London Boobies, not to menshun yer Yank F.I.B.s.*

*GUMSHOE FEETNOTE: Yer Fedrill Boorockracy of Instigation, wich used to be on the TV every week with Eefy Simple-list.

I hope the Queen wasn't too embarsed during them 100 yeer cerrymoneys when yer Mountee persented her with a horse and the darn thing kep turning its back on Roylty. Do you mind that on the TV? Yer Queen dint seem to mind it too much, even tho' she never got to look her gift horse in the mouth. But there musta bin an offal todoo after at yer Ragina Hindquarters. The Queen was a good sport about it, but she'd alreddy bin on two toors that yeer so I s'pose one more horse's ass woodn't make that much differents.

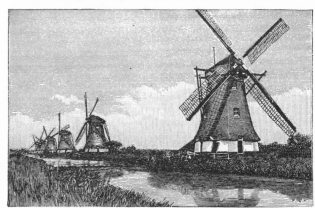

Windmill (Ragina): "We never close"

I was kinda glad to see yer Red Coat worn around agin. Used to be the only Mounted in his fantsy dress you'd git ta see round anybuddy's parts would be on the late show with that haff Nelson Eddy singing that Injian Mating Call to his other haff, Jean A. Macdonald. And it warn't too long ago that them Grits in yer Common House was trying to dress them down in brown, er even plane clothes, and cut the Rs offa them. You can still see the odd one lookin' browndoff givin' out parkin' tickets at yer airport. And some of them underware-cover ones has to go without ther clothes when they pertend to be hippos lookin' fer drug pushees sellin' yer Hishash. But I don't think our Queen wud allow them Libreeals to cut off ther insigglya and make them walk around in a uniform with jist P on it.

There's bin a lotta roomers in yer

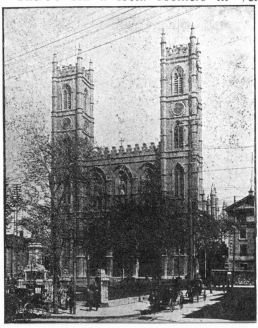

R.C.M.P. Headquatters

R.C.M.P.s this year about them fellers not bein' too happy in ther lot out in Ragina. It gits cold out there, and come Febyouary out North Battleforit way you feels the need of yer Stansfeelds balls-brigands thunderware. But accorn to the papers, yer Commissionaires won't allow ther Mounteys to have no Union soots.

It seems, too, yer Mountie wants to go into Labor. But that takes nine munths, and they got a funny rool on yer Farce that a man is not allowed to git into Holy Acrimony rite away, but has to wait two yeers fer to git dispinsensation from sumuther Supeerier Offiser. He's jist s'posed to sellabait while he waits. I dunno what he'd have to sellabait about. Mebbe yer R.C.M.P. reely stands fer yer Roamin Cathlick Munks and Preests.

I think they shood turn yer Ragina baraks into a ree-form scool. By that I mean make it By-sectional and allow yer Co-heds in. Fer why shoodn't wimmen be Mounted? Otherwise them big manly fellas'll git offal tired of celler-batin' and mebbe start up a Men's Libb. Before you know it, they'll be marchin' round outside in ther Union Suites burnin' ther jockey-straps. I don't think there's nuthin' wrong with changing yer R.C.M.P. trainin' baraks into a more Normal Scool. Let yer boys in cereese have a chants to be yuman beans . . . "on thru the hale we're a packa hungry wolves with our tail." I never did like that emblim they have up on the wall "We always gits our man." Fur a change, they deserves to git the gurl. It's helthier.

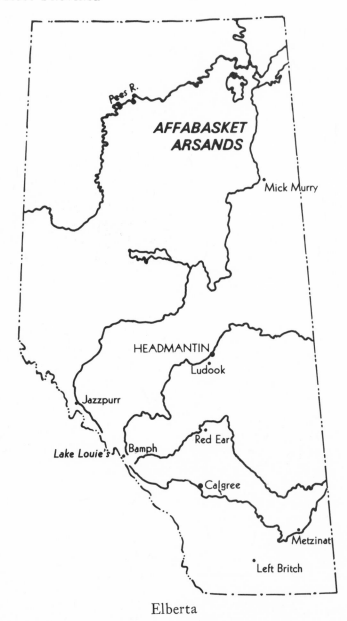

Elberta

ELBERTA

A nacheral gas of a province. Named after one of yer dotters (the peech of the crop) of the old Queen from Victoria, who marred her off to yer Markwhist FurLorne. He's the one Genrally Governed 18-78-83.*

Land: In spite of being in yer foot-ills of yer Rockys on yer rite-hand side, the place has a offal lot of good arab-bull soil. No-

*KEWBIC FEETNOTE: Them was the yeers Princess Elberta was out here from Ingaland, not her metrical messuremints.

buddy farms further north than yer frozen Pees River peeple. Yer suthernest parts is Bad Lands, semi-Arrid . . . with lots of erosenuss zones forming weerd lookin' butts and hoohoos. But ther's good valley land in yer Bow, yer Elbow, and yer Old-man Rivers, surrounded by steep bluffs so far not called by Ottawa.

Wind: Only yer Elbertans has Schnooks, a wetmass that drops its lode off over yer Rockys, then deesends on Callgary bringing warmare and turnin' yer snow-covered coolies into melting plots. It's a welcome releef (as the fella said at the cross-country busstop). But sometimes after yer ice has melt yer road to mud, that's when yer Schnook turns into yer Sch-muck.

And after they've passed that wind, the hole of Elberta becomes a skatin' rink agin and ther is grate danger to life and limb, 'speshully in yer lumber regions.

Stampeed: Ten daze that shakes the wirld. I offen wonder how they make them buckin' brontes rear up so, but they tell me it's a sinch. They got chuckle-wagging races, bulls dragging, bronchial bustin', ridin' sacred cows, and caff raping.*

Callgury is at the bend of yer Albow, wich is why yer Stampeed is sich a suck sess. The name itself is not Injian but old

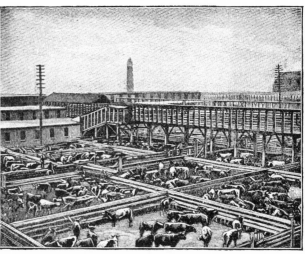
Caligari stock compny

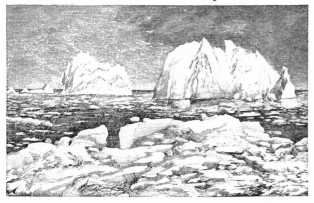
Before —

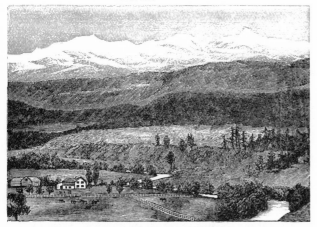
—and after yer schnook

Scotch Gay-lick. It means "cleer runnin' water" . . . but most Caligarians takes ther Elberto V.O. Fifths strait.

Clawndike Daze: After yer Stampeed is stampood out, it's yer Edmonturn. This is where the peeple, not the horses, kick up their heels. The men dress up as gay pross-peckers in ther Nineties, and the wimmen all look like gold-diggers, wearin' Asstrich feathers, er even a rhinestone Terara to match their Bum-D.A.

Nashnul Parking: Since they got more oily munny to spend on sich things, Elberta is more seenic than yer other prayery provinces. It's got lakes like Attabastard, Bitcho, Clairoil, and Utik-human . . . not to menshun Lake Louse, which is one of yer Branff Lakes I cud take every morning reglar.

They got good mountins like Mount Rumbel, wich sounds like it's soon to be vulcanized. Mount Norky is where they give you quite a lift fer to git to the top, so's you can look down in the clear air and seprate yer sheep from yer goat. There's a grate vew from Marbles Canyon, but don't look down or you mite loose yours. Also, you kin git a good peak at Bertish Clumbia thru yer Kacking Horse Piss.**

---

*LEEGLE FEETNOTE: That should be roping, but they go 'bout it much the same way.

**SPOONERD FEETNOTE: It's Kicking Horse Pass. Gonna have to watch them vowl movemints.

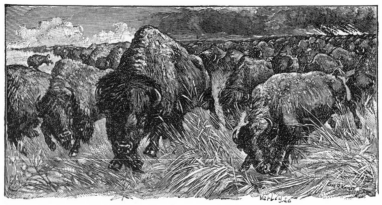

"Not as good as last year's stampeed"

Culcher: Pale-Yontology, wich is not wot I thot . . . a Histry of yer White Race . . . but turns out to be c'lectin' old bones,* and makin' a erection with them. These bones is genuwine anteeks, put together from old riptiles and made into a kinda

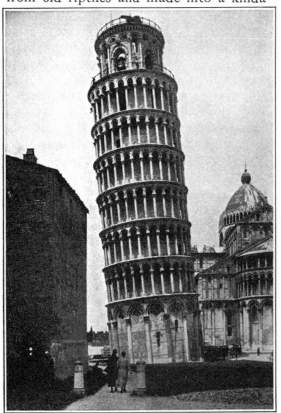

Shat-ola Comb Hotel, Edmantun

* BONEY FEETNOTE: I knew a fella before the war done that, and he never thot he was cultur'd. C'lected old bottles, too.

Dinashore show. They even look like they're forging on the grass the way they done all them peons ago. Mind you, the bones is covert over (otherwise wud look like a big turky after one of our Farquharson monster Re-union dinners). A fleet of taxidermises has got them stuffed till you'd sware you was in yer Stoned Age.

I keep wondrin' what'll happen to us Homeo saplings when we start to extink. Mebbe the cockaroaches will do the same fer us when we end up as the skelton in our own closet.

Mine In: Not too much outside of yer Peter-out-chemcals. Elberta cole is the coke kind, and the Jap seems to think things go better with it because he's jist shipped a lot off to his land of the rising slum.

Japs seem to like Canda. I gess they got used to it during the war when we put them into Nissein huts in yer constipation camps. That was after they changed yer U.S. navels base at Perl's Harber into a musuleum fer stationery submarines.

I mind reeding in the paper, I think it was yer *Meaford Suppository*, about some Jap that had bin hidin' out in the fathills and jist give hisself up when he reelized the war was over. When he seen all them Datsums and To-yoyos twixt Edmington and Caligari with their Panicsonic stereeo raddios, he jist natcherly figgerd Canda was pree-occewpied with Japan winning the war. And, by gol, I don't think he was so fur off.

Oil: Is wot has moved Elberta out of yer Aggra-arian Econmy into yer Plutocraps. This is nothin' to do with Mickey Mice's dog. It's wot yer rich oilmen plays when they hed fer Loss Wages, Nevadder.

It's not too easy to throw up yer oil like they done at LeDook in '47. Oil is found in dome-shaped fermations like yer Hoostom Asterdoom or Rakels Welk. Nowadays, they starts by gittin' foty-grafts from a satlight circumcising the erth. Nex', they git closer-ups with a helluvacopper. Then it's into yer bush with yer packhores. A core drill (not yer army manoovers but a puntable rig mounted on a Mac's truck) is nozzled into yer ground fer to brake the old rocks off and bring up yer first Samples. If yer junior Samples looks good, then yuh gits past all that old shist of yer sheeld and down to the Basil Conglummerate, down between the sheets of bedrock. 'Tween the sheets is yer slates of shale. Problem is fer to git the shale out of there.

Out of 1700 hole that's bin well-drilled since '68, only 580 come up oily . . . 350 was gassy . . . and the rest come up dryer'n the teats on a bull. Sometimes with yer cyclic carbonates* you gits no stratus-faction from yer inter-fingering. And when yer sillycones starts to sag, then you've blew the hole thing syncline and hooker.

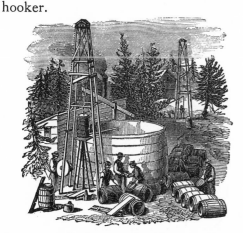

Refinement in Alberta

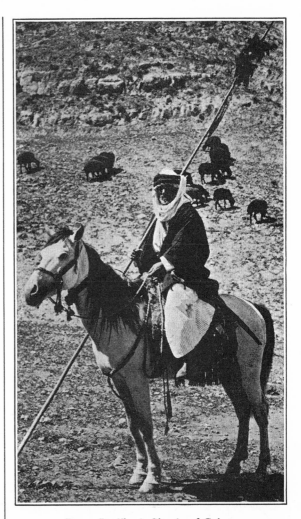

Peter Luffhed, Sheek of Calgry

It took more'n twenty years of dry holes around Edmington before they blew LeDook. Wot Elbertins is waiting for in future is to lick the tar out ther sands. But they have to figger a way to git the Grits out first. A new Sinkrude plant will cost 400 millyun, not includin' yer carrying charges piping it to Edmonturn. When the whissle blows on that, it shood replace Marg Lalonde** as Canda's biggest pli-tickle football.

It costs money to be yer oily bird, becuz oil is not like yer Hydra, wich kin be used over and over retractably. But Elbertans don't seem to go in fur yer 'lectrics so

*LO-CAL FEETNOTE: Orville sez that must be yer Tab and yer Fresky.

**PIGSKIN FEETNOTE: Them two Bassetts, yer John and yer Junior, found out Lalonde is Strong.

much. I gess they 'member us Ontaryans fer the nite we blacked out the hole of yer Uppa Ewe Ass when we bloo the fews on our Queenston Jennyrater. It was only one nite, but nine months later yer Land of yer Free and Eazy had a copulation explosion.

So Elbertans don't trust too much to yer Easterer. 'Speshully Donald McDonald, who'se tried everything (he's bin hed of yer Steal Workers, a big wheel in yer CCM, and with yer Canadyan Congers in Labor), and now he's the Minster without the Energy to Mind Our Resources. But he's had sevral gass attacks from Peter Luff-hed, who give him the Shakes of Calgeree.

You mind last winter when Macdonald was trying to do somethin' fer our nashnul unititty by gettin' us all to turn out the lites and go to bed erly? (And by gol, if that don't bring us together, nothin' will.) The idee was to get us all to cut back our energy ten purscent. The example was set by yer Ottawa Shrivelled Service, who'd bin doin' jist that fer the past 20 yeer. But it warn't yer Allergy crisis at all. It was jist them harem-scarem Shoddy Arapians razing ther prices. As soon as we pade ten cents a gal more, the hole shor-tidge dispeered quicker'n yer Comet Ko-hotex.

I'll say one thing fer yer hed of Imperious Oil, W. O. Twits. He was honist enuff to admit he was awreddy doin' pritty good, even before they tacked on that extra sixty cents a barl. (If he ever leaves his remanes to posteerior, I'd sure love to have his Gaul.) It seems to me he was the smart one and we're the twits. I think I may jist git a poortrait of him in oil fer Chrissmus, sints he's alreddy done me in gas.

Mind you, I don't blame them West-erers fer charging more after wot we've bin doin' to them with yer frate rapes. And it's hardly gonna put them into yer Transports of delight when yer Minster in Charge of Railin', Jene Merchant (in French that'd be Jong Mah-jong), jist wipes his hands and throws up.

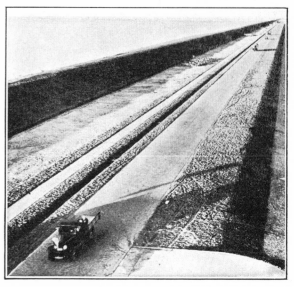

Libral cockus on the move

You cud see the results in yer last 'lection. Even tho' Mistair Trudo fin'ely attained his majorty (and at his age!), all the Libreeals in Alberta blew ther deposits.* Elberta is now a Sepertist state, Bob Stansfeeld has sed Farewell and Hailo to Novy Skosher, and they say Medzin' Atters is startin' to bild the little log cabin little Jack Corner was borned in. And Pierre Trudo is now payin' tenshun to yer West. No more dancing with yer Red squares in Mascow, or skinny dipping in the Bertish Houndyerass. Pee-air has got his hed to the grindstone now, hoping that when he asts the West to lower ther prices, they won't say back to him, "Up Yores!"

But I think the West's mane complaint agin Ottawa was callin' that 'lection on Elberta's holyday, yer openin' of yer Stampeed. You talk about a dry hole—that was Calgry last July 8. That'd be the day yer Seprators moved from Cue-bec West.

Curling: Besides yer oil, another big occupayshun out west is curling up fer the winter with yer broom-mate and brakin' the wind in front of yer stones. It's all ammerchewers in yer curling, jist ornery

*POLITICKLE FEETNOTE: Orville wonders why they made so much fuss over two cents on the bottle.

peeple tryna make ther Big Ends meat. But wherever two er three Eldbertens gathers together on ice, you got a Bumspeel. Now, there's them as sez yer Nashnul's sport is LaCrotch. (That's gang whorefare plaid by them warped racketeers.) But I bleeve yer Injians was curlin' as well as lacrotchin' before yer white man cum. How elts did them Stonied Injians git ther name? Er yer Backfeet? I ast Cheef John Snow* at the Injian Mewseum at Morley if his tribe wasn't swinging ther stones long before we moved in. He sez his bunch razed a wick er two, but them Schnooks come along agin from B.C. and changed the name of yer game to water poolo.

Wich minds me, I dunno what yer Injians wore when they slid on ther draws.

*CHEEF FEETNOTE: John got his last name from the kinda job the guvmint has been givin' him fer yeers. One of the fellas got a step-up las' summer when he were made 'Tennant Guvnor, with reservayshuns.

Mebbe a loinin cloth. Yer Scot used to ware his kilt, until he got the wind up. Now he jist keeps a little tassole on his tammyshatner in mammary of yer Blue-Balls of Scotland.

Elberta won yer Bryer last year . . . yer Bryer, that'd be Canda's biggest Rock Festerall . . . and the hole thing was skipped by Hec Dervish, a whirl of a potato farmer who'd Tabored down a few pounds since he'd bin one of yer former Tit-lists in '61. I seen yer Elbertans win myself down there to London hard by St. Thomas. Premeer Billy Davis was there to do yer openin' cerrymonial. He was ast to cast the first stone jist to prove he was without sin amongst us. But the fella I wanted to see in action on that ice was Preenyer Terdo, fer he to me is yer hed of yer perfect set of cerlers . . . you jist watch the sweeping statemints he makes as he skips every issyuh.

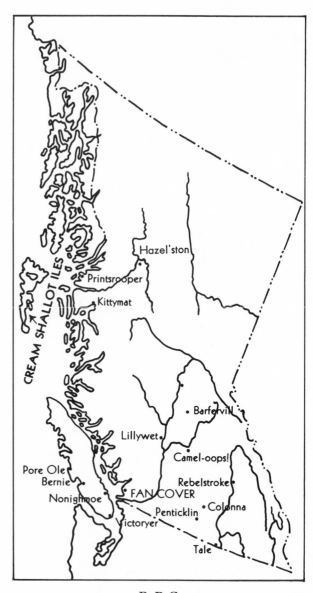

B. B. C.

B.B.C.* YER MOUNTIN PAIRADICE

The mutto in pig-Lattin is "SPLENDOR SINE OCCASU," wich when dun up in Anglish by yer Loose translater seems to be "IT NEVER WANES BUT IT SPLINTERS."

Yer Coat-with-Arms has got a lion standing abuve yer old flag we used to have, and yer flag is sittin' on yer sun settin' in the water. This used to meen yer Bertish Umpire going down fer the last time on yer Impress Hotel in Victorier, but has laitly come to meen yer Rising Son comin' up on yer Union Jap. Watching all this on eether side of yer Sheeld is yer two Nachuralized B.C.ers, yer toothy Elk and yer Mounted Sheep.** (I think it was yer Flyin' fishy Fill Jellardy who divided yer popillation into his Sheep and his Goats, but times has changed.)

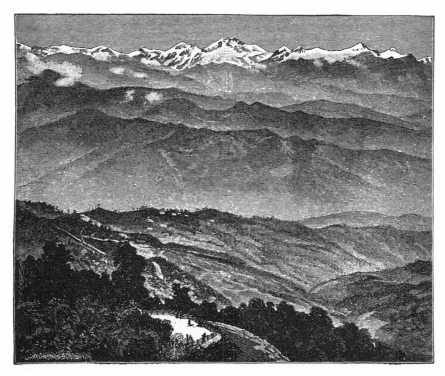

The Grannit Curtin

Top-Hogriffy: Altho' not as broad as she's long (760 mile up and down, and mebbe 400 mile acrost . . . give er take 50 mile fer to git yer Rockys off), B.C. stretches from yer Alastcan Panhandlers rite down b'low yer boarder into yer Straits of Wanta Fewcup.

You talk about variety bein' yer change of life, B.C. is yer place. Mix yer Norweejin Ford with yer Serf of Callfornya and throw in a bit of yer Crotchswolled Hills in Old Ingaland, pluss Cue Gardens up yer Tems and yer Swish Alps, and mebbe by then yule git some idee of Bertish Clumbya. It must be tuff tryna cut down a tree wen you got one foot up a mountin' and the t'other one suckin' in yer wet sand. But that's B.C., and yer lokels say you gotta like it or limpit.

Climbit: Jist dendy if you likes topickal rane forsts. Talk about yer inter-mitten reesipitating, it can happen anywears anytime. I've herd of peeple gittin' cot in Standley Park with nothin' between them and the ground but ther feeancey.

If yer like me and like to be in seesin, you won't git too much differents in B.C. between yer Equinux. Yer leef don't give you much of a turn, and you don't notice yer fall comin' on till yer folyage starts to drop off. But it's milder on accounta they import mosta ther whether currantly from Japan. They send over the North Specifick Drift fer to keep the warm water on tap a tall times. Mind you, once in a wile, yer Coaster don't git the drift, but mostly yer hole province is now run by yer Japaneeze currancy.

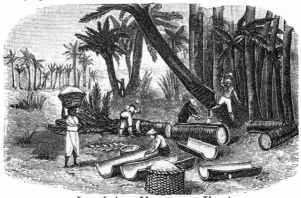

Lumbring, Vancoover Iland

Yer Mounts: First thing yer Vankoovrite points to you outa his kitchin window is that they all have quite a range. Only trubble with sich a high stand of rock is it gits in the way of yer vew. It's on accounta yer Rocky and yer Sellquirks that one haffa yer provinshuls don't know how them other haff lives. All that mountin seenery is divissif. Yer highest you git is Mount Farewether (wich is named after a lokel Vancoover joke).

It's on accounta the mountins that three quarts of yer Resdants lives on only five purrsent of yer land, eether coastal strippers or furtle Vallyeers up yer interior, wher they lives pritty strung out all the time. Even tho' they don't seem at home on yer ranges, they must hit the peeks with wat they do in between, fur yer popillation has tripletted since yer last wore. Valeda, the wife and former sweethart, she thinks it's all that skeejumpin' that's to blame . . . fer after they git all the way down them hills and kick ther slats off, they jist gotta do somethin' to wile away the time.

Favrit places fer girl watches is Mount Whistler, and favrit place to complane about not havin' any girls to watch wud be yer Grouse Mountin. And them she-skeers that gits preggerunt is confined to Mount Waddlingtun. If you go by yer berth raight, looks like after-the-shee is yer provinshul's favrit indore sport. Sept in summer, when they all put ther little dingys in the water.

Forsts: Ya'd think it was yer mountin is the backbone of this place, but it's yer Duggle-ass fur. The offishul flour of B.C. is yer Dogwould, and no one is aloud to raze a hand agin it . . . or foot (speshully dogs).

The mane pree-ockipation . . . apart from propagaiting . . . wud be log-rolling, axe-ing, and saw-offs. (I'm not jist talkin' about yer Guvmint, what have told many a sittizen to go clime a tree.) Yer biggest pulphouse is MacMilkin-Blowedhell, and they're cookin' mosta the time, sept last yeer when they was struck by the fack

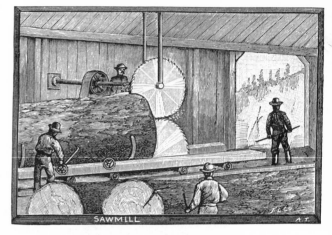

Duglass Fur Storage

that ther wooden workers wooden work.

Furs: Not yer Duggle-ass kind, but yer hoof 'n claw. Sum furs is farmed out, like yer chinchilla is razed (purty much the same way as minks do it). But mosta yer hairy ones runs wild up northa Prints Gorge. (I ment aminals, but the peeple has a pretty good time, too.) Most faimuss of yer B.C. wild animal is sort of a Abdominal Snowman called yer Suskwatch, kind of a haff-bare man stands hire than yer Graycups Goaly post. He hasn't yet bin captivated, but a good livin' can be made sellin' his footprints to

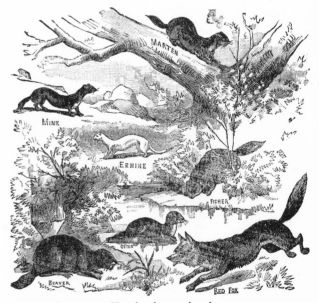

Fer boring animals

nudespapers like yer *Nashnul Inkwirer*, yer *Hash*, and yer *Flush*.

Fission: I don't mean yer Nukuler, altho' that's what they was worryed about cuppla yeers ago when the Yanks was lettin' off a couple big bomms up Amchitkicker way. Yer *Greenpeas* boat went up to see if ther was any fall-off (wot they call in syentifickle terns yer Playhouse 90), but now everybuddy is wurried about yer spill-off from yer oil slickers out of yer Alaskacans.

them whine. (Some of the whinin' comes from Ontaryo's Nagger Escrapmint, wher they don't want nuthin' to compete with ther Bright's future.)

Grane: Everything must be aginst the grane. Only two purcent of yer land is arrible! Yer Frazure Valley has a nice dairy air, and up in yer top rite hand corner is a Peece where wheet's groan. I dunno how they keep yer Peece warm that fur up, but they grows yer Markus weet, wich keeps hard without too much smut.

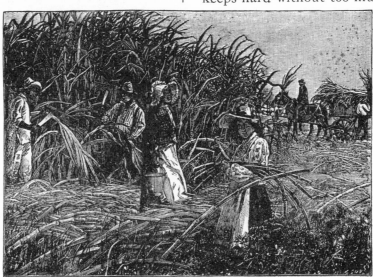

Yer Peece Score

But slick er not, yer sammon is still the catch of the seesin, on accounta it's one fish that'll go to any lengths fer to git laid . . . even clime ladders. I dunno what aigs them on, but they jist haff to git back fer Old Home week. And mosta them when they gits ther is too tuckert out to do nothin' but drop the hole thing.

Froot: Yer Oaken Noggin is secund only to Ontaryo in yer froot abun-dance, and ther apples is Delishus to ther corps. Mosta yer froots is deported in pritty good condishun, sept that them as isn't froze is smudged. **Vermin** (on accounta all the trees its infesterd with) and **Pintickling** (named after yer motel mat-tresses) are both packed with froots in seesin, wile **Killowner** takes them froots and makes

Meet: A lotta cattle is renched up in yer Carryboozer's country and stuffed on the spot. But sum is sent to finshing scools in Elberta (I bin force-feeding my boy Orville fer yeers) and packed home agin to yer local cutter-upps.

Mini-rails: Is wat started the hole thing. Even before Conflagration, Yale men was tryna git to Bartervill to trade ther soles fer gold. Not much gold left, but if you wanna git the led out, try **Kim Berly**. Or if you likes assbestus, check yer Casheers mountins. **Kittymat** was chose as yer best box-site and it pro-juices Hydro as well as illuminatum. (As well as rooning yer Tweedsmanure Nashnul Parking Spot.*) In yer Kootenannies jist off

*WET FEETNOTE: But do they care? Not by a dam site.

yer Trail is yer biggest smeller. Yer Comin-go peeple are proving that every zink has a silver lining . . . and they know how to distract it.

Reck-creation: The biggest bizness of all in B.C. is flappin' ther gums about how lucky youse are to be there. They make it sound like You-top-ya, and tooryists come from as neer away as Oargone and Warshinton . . . A.C.D.C. (Acrost from Canda, Down yer Clumbya). Them loose livers like our floatin' doller. Mind you, yer lokels spends ther halldays in Hwyee or Acapello, Maxico. They say ther jist tryna git away frum all them dust-bowellers from Saskachewin.

One thing I'd like to see is all them nudee-ist camps, where you can see fer yerself that things reely swing.

Vancoozer: Canda's biggest outdoors port, thanks to yer Robbers Bank, and the home of sum of our best indoor sports. They got more culchur than pencil-linen . . . more sympathy orchesters than you kin shake a stick at. Always looking fer house-room, it's sumtimes called Van-

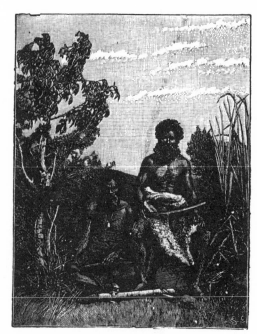
Gassed Towners

couver BP on accounta yer Bertish Propreyeitties still owns mosta yer mountin-sites since Captin Crook first landed ther.

Yer eldest part of Vancoozer was called Gassed Town and it's now divvied up between yer Hippos and yer Gorgeous Straits. The rest of yer animals is in Stanely Park (named after the grassmarks on yer knees). But nuthin' ever gits dirty out here becuz yer daly rane washes

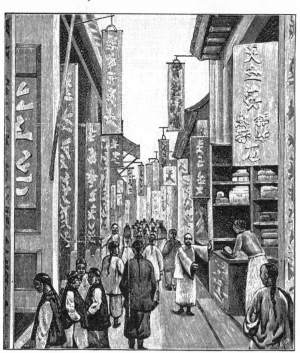
Downtown Fang Coover

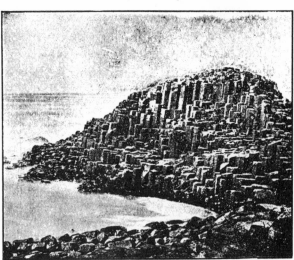
Hyrize at Anglish Bay

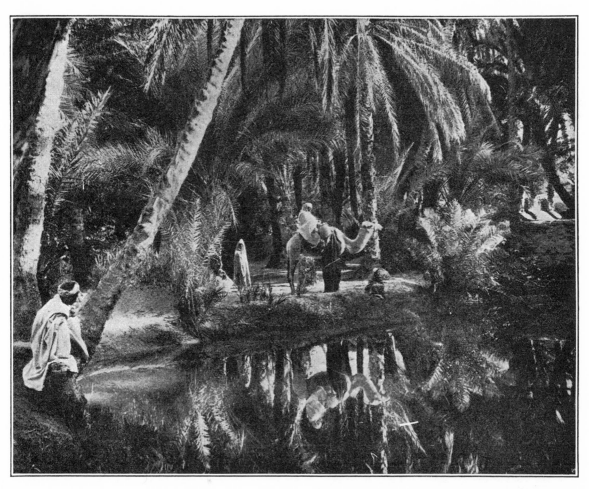

Yer Conserve-a-tory, Impress Hotel, Victoria,   B.C.

everythin' cleen, wich is probly why they call yer downtown arear Shinytown, my Shinytown. One or t'other side of Lion's Gate Bridge (bilt with the money from Foot Ball Games) is yer sublerbs of Newest Minister, Burnybee, Wes Van, Horseshad Bay . . . and they has got more swim-in pools than yer entire Prayery provins has in weet. Howe Sound yer econmee is I dunno. Never know when you mite get a chilly wack frum yer Ottawa vallee. In case that happens, Vancoozer is the home of "See Pee-Air," a airline that takes you rite to 24 SubSex Drive, home of our luvly Prime Mistress, Margrit.

Prince Rupee: Another athletic seaporter, and yer Skeeny river makes it easy to Terrass down to Kittymat. Up river is **Hazel'ston,** wher they keep all yer token poles to Pacificfy yer Shimshams and yer Kwackydoodle into accepting them tall tellyphone rates.

Victorius: The pote sed, "No man's land is an Iland." But then he hadn't took a ferry over and seen the sites of **Pore Erl Bernie, Ninnynymo,** and **Skymalt,** wher yer Royl Rodes scullers scabs the deck.

The old Victorians lives down at the bottom of the ile by the Birdcages. All them dubble-dipper buses is lined up in front of yer Impress Hotel in case sumbuddy ever comes out. I ast one old feller what he was waiting fer in yer lobbly, and he sed, "George! the Fifth!" Turned out it was a waiter with a bottle.

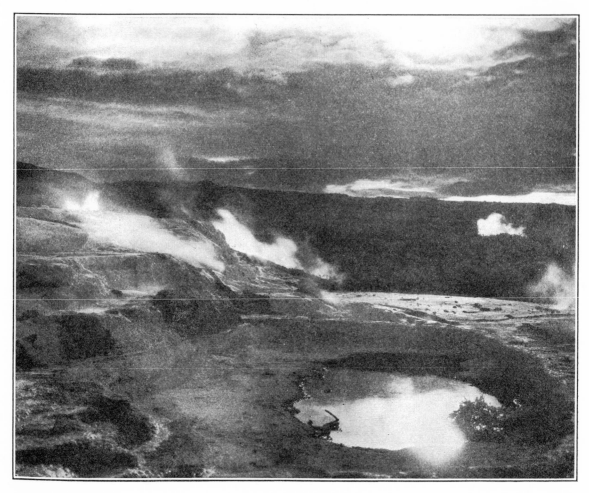

Harassing Hot Springs

But Victoria is rabid with sum of its groath. Yer Cent-a-nennial Mozleum is next to yer Hotel. (Why they want a mozleum when they got that hotel is sumthin' I'll never unnerstand.) And yer Arch Hives is next to that, but I don't think there's bin much of a swarm goin' in so far. Next to that is yer Birdcage, wich was not too long ago cleened out and a new rooster put in.

Guvmint: He's yer big, broad, ruggered and rotunda Dave Bart. He's the N.D. Pier tuk over from yer Sociable old Credit Card Whacky Benny.*

*RE-TIRED FEETNOTE: Reel name is R. B. Benny and he was Premeer in his 30's ever since we all had the big depressyun. R.B. stands for Rithm And Booze, both of wich he wud have none of.

Dave he's a big bluff, harty kinda gink who kin take a joke along with the rest of them. (And by golly so kin the rest of them, or they wud never have 'lected him in the first place.) Since he's bin sittin' in yer Birdcage, everybuddy sure knows he's bin there, becuz a big bird like Dave as soon as he finds his perch likes to swing a little. He's ruffed a few of the sitty feathers, but his mane trubble has bin in Labor. He'd no sooner got into his offiss than ther was that strike on the iland at the hite of yer Toorist Seesin. Peeple was lined up fer forty ate hours, tryna sleep in ther Folkswaggins. Well sir, Dave he went down to yer water's edge and ordered them Murine capt'ns to take them cross toorists over from Youclueless to Squeamish. Did they budge? You jist ask Dave Bart if he bleeves any more in ferrys.

Dave's had a lotta more trubble with his water. He's bin tryna rechoke the agreemint that old Whacky made fer to let the entire providence drip down to the States come Hail Clumbia er highwater. You'd think them Yanks wud git enuff run-off jist from yer Law of Gravelty workin' its way down. But a wile ago them Oargoners at Point Robbers, hard by yer Pewkit Sound, made sich a stink about not havin' enuff that Dave Bart got NDPeed off enuff to thretten to cut ther water off.

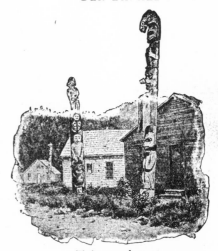
Token poles

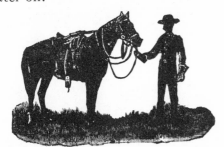
Silooet in Lilooet

I dunno why yer Yank feels he has to make a grab at our assets, sints they got us purty much encircle-sized by now, and all they has to do is clip the coopons. Mind you, Dave Bart's got idees about them ownin' us lockstock and over-yer-barl. He's one of yer more promnint Sociable-ists, alwayz out in yer four-front (if you take a good look at him from the side). And he's after the private sextor

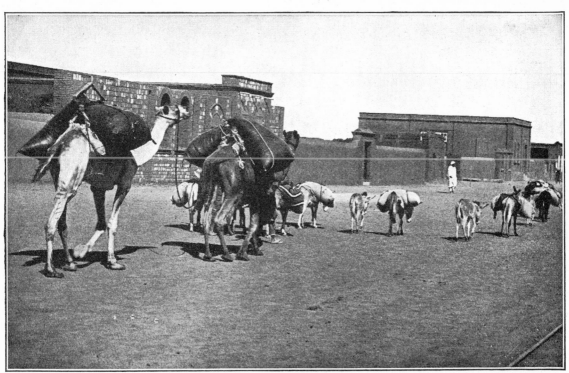
Camel-oops!

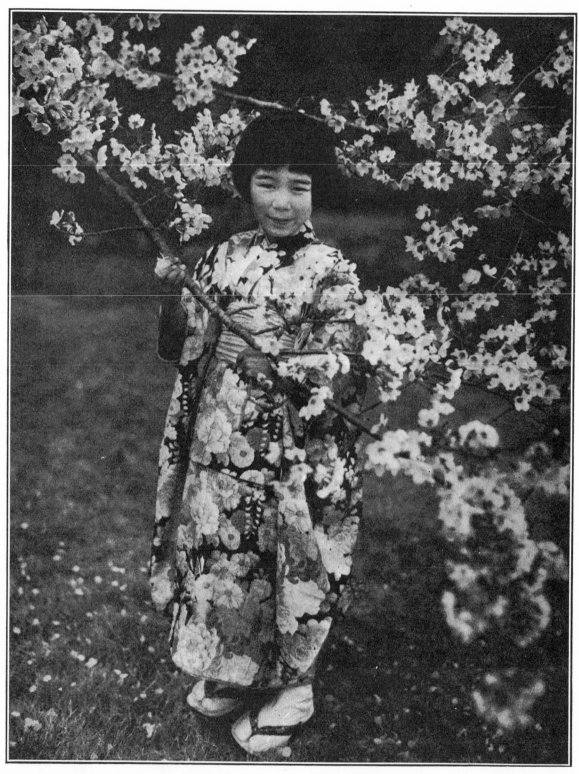

Maid in Japan, invests in B.C.

of all yer B.C. econmee. He's done it alreddy with yer otto insurience thru no fault of his own. He's started his own Bank, becuz one of his 'lection promissorys was "You kin bank on Dave." And next he'll be takin' on yer pulpy peeple becuz Dave he can't leeve them lagers alone. Do you mind the time yeer before last he went out with yer fishy fleet? Him and his hole cabnet got tuk on bored (sept fer that Cabnet member that got lopped off fer presenting his breefs in the back of a car), and all them M.P.P.s was squished into gumboots and southwesterners till they looked like an Ad fur Scotch Repulsion. They had a fine time halling in somebody else's line fur a change, and by yer weak-end they was all mooching fur Colehole sammon jist like a buncha happy hookers. (Probly took home mosta yer net profits too, if I know them guvmint fellas.)

I think it's a darn good idee fer offisuls that looses touch with yer Commner people to git out and do some work for a livin'. I woodn't mind havin' a few of them cleen out my barn. Becuz them Cabnet fellers is experks . . . they bin spreddin' that stuff around fer yeers.

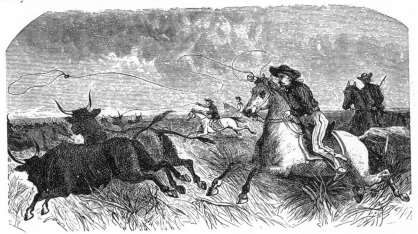

Carrypoo cowpokers

YER UKE-ON: CANDA'S GHOSTAL ZONE

Yer Uke-on is the skelton in Canda's closet, havin' took only seventy yeer fur to become so pree-histerical.

It jist never got over its first rush ($18.98) during yer Clowndike Stampeed (wich sounds like a combine week-end in Calgree and Edmington, but was reely a big strike fur gold). But yer ores soon becum all worked out, and yer sourdose all went back to the States to seattle down. If yer cheef expork was gold at that time, yer cheef impork was cans of beens . . . and by gol ever one of them is still there rustycating.*

Yer Uke-on is not so much growed-up as growed-over. On accounta yer high frate rates, nothin' was ever returnable. It was jist last spring that they finely got around to kicking the last can offa yer war-time Highway that has the same name. It was in '42 that yer Lastcan root was bilt becuz yer Yanks thot the Japs had alleutions about evading us, or bomming the Amchitkikas out of us with ther Komicrazy pilot pogrom run by Harry Carey. So yer U.S. and us co-opulated in driving this cordyal rode from Dawesome to Whitehores. And every-body went truckin' on down till VD day, when they all went home with ther dis-charge and left yer Hyway to the Moose and the Mariboo sniffing amongst yer emtee Spamcans.

Industree: Here the Guvmint is yer Mr. Big. It's the closest thing Canda's got to yer well-fired state. But a toorist Hazin is wat yer Uke-on is turnin' on to be. They was jist flooded with them this summer (and the vicey of yer versey, wich put a damper on ther things!). But everybuddy wants to see the place wher Charlie Chaplin et his shew at the big end of yer Chiclet Pass. They wanna see wher Jack London stuck it out with his White

*CLEEN FEETNOTE: The guvmint has promised to cleen the hole place up so's Pee-Air Berton can bring his kids back fer another visit. Too bad 'Liz can't come along too. But Miss Taylor and he have splitt upp.

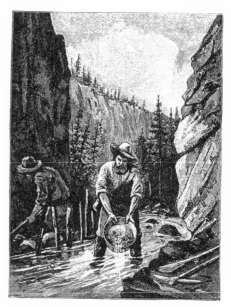

Looking fer berried goldwater

Fangs, and Robert's Service Station wher he writ about "The Creeatin of Mike Magee" and "Dangerous Dan Magoo at yer Lady's Loo."

You talk about yer litter-airy remanes, yer Yukon got lots all over. It looks like a Jumbled White Elfint Sail to wich no-buddy ever come. Even them big dredges, what come bullsdozing in after yer rush fer to git out what gold was left, is still there up at Bananza Crick. (This is nuthin' to do with yer TV Banaanzais with yer Cartweel famly hedded up by Ponderose Lorngrin.) Be funny if yer dredges brung in more gold from yer curious toorsts than all the old creaks what was dug into.

Lotsa more 'tractions fer Outlanders ta see. Yer Tuckheeny Hot Springs is a steemy place fer peeple who sulfer from yer roomytoid arthuritis. It sounds like a Motel with the Magic Fingers, but it's jist a natcherl Jackoozie whirlpool givin' off a sike-opathic massage.

One of the bigger 'tractions is yer drinking laws. Sort of a "whut-the-heck let-it-all-hang-over" altitude. 'Stedda sayin' "If you drink don't drive," yer Mounty jist says "As long as yer not impaired, you won't git impeeched." It don't seem to make no differnts to the number of drunks, but it sure cuts down on the howzing problem in yer who'sgow.

Gold: Now that the wirld is back on yer Gold Standerd Time, they mite git a second rush up yer Chilly-cool Passage. It seems that gold is cremated by yer vulcanic peece of ash boilin' over, gittin' froze by yer ice, and ground down by yer sand rite in the nuggets. This happens when yer erth tilts a lot, and yer Uke-on since it started has bin one big pinballs masheen. So mebbe yer minor shud give it anuther whirl. Lotsa arn ore lying around on top of the ground, but ther'sa reeson you can't git it to market. That's no ship, b'leeve me.

There's lotsa old stern-weelers sittin' around on ther bottoms cud git steemed up agin, but sum fool injunear has bilt his britches too low acrost yer Uke-on river fer yer well-stacked scow. That's the trubble with yer Roads scoller. They'll bild a square bridge that won't come unhinged and swing a little. 'Stoo bad, fer you can't beet bein' paddled by yer old sternweeler.

Furs: Worn by bares, brown, black, grisly, and kodak. But I don't advise nobuddy to try to take ther coats off, less you want a fite to yer finnish.

Farm: Short groan sessin—less'n two

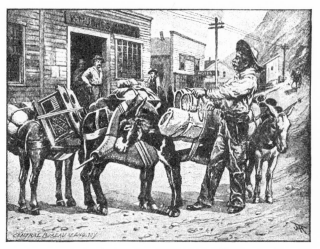
Packin' 'em in at Dawsome Sitty

month—but it's a 22-hour day and gives you cabbitches big as sockerballs and collyflours like waggin weels. But wood you bleeve there's only one workin' farm in yer hole terrtory? And even that's endanger of oil prosspeckers 'cause farmers got no rites, speshully minral rites, and anybody can stake a claim thru them.

But yer native's peeple is startin' to fite back. The ones next door in Lasker hired a brace of white lyers and won a settlmint offa yer Capital's Dome in Warshinton of a billyun dollers. Fer that kinda munny, all yer native foke cud retire to yer Hy-wayin Ilands and live on the Dole with pine-apples.

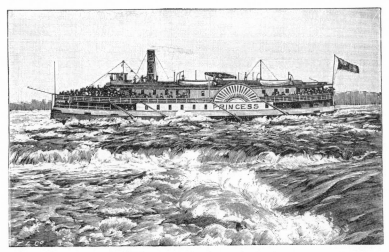
Old-time rapids transit, You-Kon

Dawsum: (Pop 12,000)* There used to be as manny peeple here round yer tern of yer sentry as is now in the hole of yer North from Pointa Barrow to Bafflin Iland. Now, it's a curious kind of town with three museums and probly more to come . . . but not to stay.

Whitehores: Yer other anker point at the t'other end of yer All-can Highway. Also has a rale on with Scragway, Alaskher.

Climbact: Yer climaxtick condishuns is the limit. Jist remember Joon is spring and Awgist is Autum. And in between is where yuh gits yer first frost . . . and that's a bad place to git it.

Future: It looks like yer Yukon will soon be dammed. Yer power-peeple wanna yoke yer U-con River and make it flow back t'other way. Like the ad sez, it's not nice to fool with Mother's nature, and yer dam ain't natcheral. It bloats up yer lakes, trickelates yer rivers, muds up yer flats, and drowns yer tree, jist like they done in B.C. with them ded logs lying all over yer Kittymat.

Yer white man thinks he's bringin' in sumthin' speshul. Last time he dun that it was yer inflewensa. He brung the flu in and then flu out . . . and left yer natives coffin' up ever sints.

*DRUGGED FEETNOTE: That's peeple, not pills.

Youcon roots + froots +gourd only nose wat

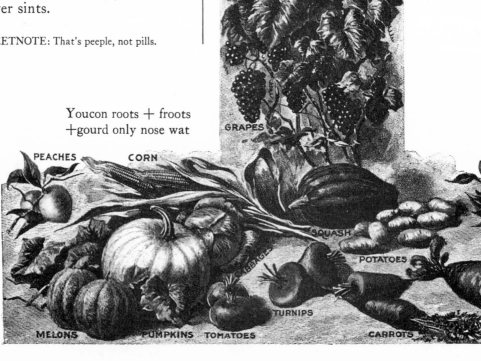

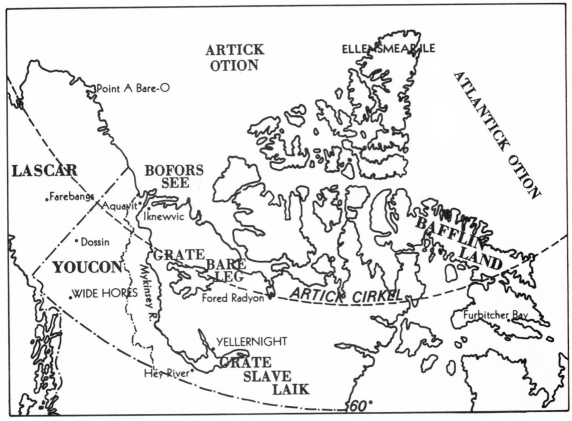

ARTICK OTION

ELLENSMEAR ILE

ATLANTICK OTION

Point A Bare-O

LASCAR

BOFORS SEE

Farebangs

Aquavit

Iknewvic

Dossin

YOUCON

GRATE BARE LEG

BAFFLIN LAND

WIDE HORES

Mykinsey R.

Fored Radyon

ARTICK CIRKEL

Furbitcher Bay

YELLERNIGHT

Hey River

GRATE SLAVE LAIK

60°

Yer Youcon and North Waste Terrortory

YER NORTH WASTE TERRORTORY: OUR FROZE ASSET

Used to be called Rooper's Land, becuz explorters serched up here fer yer northwest passidge to Injer and all them roopees. But with yer curnt developments, yer Injian and Eskmoe is starting to call it Raper's Land. Fer underneeth all this friggidititty is a lotta fossil fools.

But on the serfiss it's just barn land, a big frozen dessert with snow and icing that don't hardly ever go away . . . and that incloods yer garbitch on top of it.

Yer North Waste covers yer mainlined from yer U-con over near as fur's LoneGreeneland, pluss all the eyelands of yer Artick Archyerbellygo. That's one thurd of all the arrear of Canda and more'n twicet big as Alasky, wich is bigger'n Taxes. Wich is mebbe why alot of thim Suthern Comferters wanders up our way with ther oil rigs fer to make a few dallas. So far, yer avrage iglue has made a farely comfortable tax shelter.

Climactick: Exscream. Most of yer natives lives above ther treeline, wich leeves them exposed all yeer. In summers yer murkry gits up to mebbe 50 or 60 degree Fairinheat. But don't try to sonbath or whordes of muskeeters will give you that pebblegrane look of a pare of Dax. Springs and falls is meen rather than temprit. And winters, my gol, they'd freeze the vows offa brass munk.

Wild Life: I meen outside, with yer animal, whut's left of them . . . polerbare, carboo, seeledmeet, yer whitey and yer redd foxx. 'Twas yer whitey that got yer Eskmoe fer to trap yer fox, until the ladees had no eyes for them and they fell offa yer hat prade.

Even yer carboo is not herd so much. That riter fella with the sporrin on his

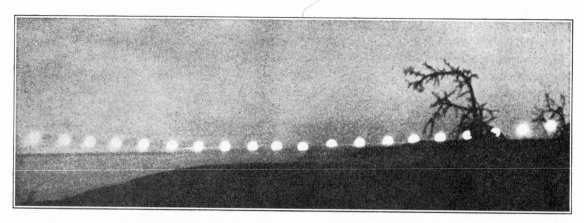

Like Orville, yer midnite son stays up all nite

face, Furry Mowit, he wants to bring raindear over from Sibeeryier and have them git milked by yer Eskymoe (fer a change). It'd be eesy to stash the empty pales ther so well hung with antleers, but I think yer avrage Esky wud jist as soon go off on a Muskrat Rambel.

Peeple: Eskmoes call therselves INNER-WITS becuz, dispite us wite men, they've maniged to keep ther sensa yuma. Ya mite be s'prised to lern that yer native is in his minnerority in his own land by now. Purrsentage wize, it's 19 Injian, 37 Eskymoe, and 44 whites. At first it was only a few bushed pile-its, but lately yer white suthern speckle-laters has brung in sich lucksurees as sedgergated beer parlers.

Yer Injian (Dogrid, Chipawayon, and Slavey) labers close to yer provinshul boarders, whereas yer Eskmoe is mostly coasters. Yer Injian gides fly-in-fishin' weakenders dippin' ther flys into yer Grate Bare Lake. They tell me the fish bites up there 24 hours a day and so does everything elts. It's no place fer them shoo-stringy Bitkeenys worn by yung floppers.

Yer Eskymo, too, goze after murine life, and they get some tasty Artick fish like yer chard and yer grayline. But they've stopped chawin' on the odd bare shoulder and started snackin' on our kinds of fud . . . choclit bars and Krackernut and ptater chippies . . . so ther startin' to git bad teeth and pimples and overwate jist like yer avrage teeny-ager. Yer Eskymoe looks round, but that don't make thim fat . . . that's jist Faceyal Discrimnation.

Artz and Crap: Nowadaze most Eskmo hunters is workin' fulltime fer yer Fed guvmint cuttin' up sope into stones. And they has terned out to be quite some cut-ups. Eskmoe carping is poplar.

Cussdem: Not much left of yer old terd-ishun. Mosta yer Eskys is adappleting to yer Grate White Way of Life. Now they take yer Old Age Penchant and keeps the grandpairnts, 'stedda puttin' them on ice until it's time fer them to floe.

But yer Eskmoe was way ahead of us in his sistern of Famly Allowances, wich he calls Wives Wopping. This has bin tuk up by us in a big way. First time I herd about it was last year, when them two Newyork perfessional ballers what had

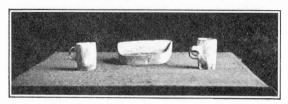

Eskmo hand mill fer crushing ice

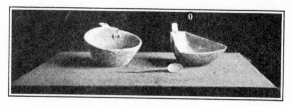

Eskmo ice mill fer crushing hands

bin releefin' eech other on yer mound started releefin' offa yer mound, too. Then, by golly, if we din't heer about the same yoke-switchin' happenin' up our way after a thrashing party this summer. Afffter a lotta drinkin', they all throo ther keys in the middle of the floor and everybuddy went home in sumbuddy elt's tractor. First thing we noo, two lokel cupples had switched ther britching and started forgin' wher they thot yer furaway grass was greener. And this four-on-the-floor bizness is still goin' on. So fur, nyther of the two partees has communy-eye-icated with t'other. But I betcha it won't be long before the one cupple will phone t'other, becuz them two wimmen must be dyin' to find out how the two men is gittin' along cookin' fer eech other.

Producks: Mane thing they got up there is yer ice and snow . . . but they don't deliver. Don't laff. Sum Americans wud like to deport it down to ther Arrid states so's they cud irritate themselves. Mind you, our water, like our beer, may be too strong fer the Yanks, and they may have to diloot it first. If there's one thing we make in Canda, it's water. Last spring I mind yer Lake Untarryo got the overflows when that little Mare Crumby told all yer develpers to go jump in the lake.

Producks-To-Be: That's what interests yer bizness tightcoons. That's why ther all up in yer Articks now checking yer gas and yer oil under that moss and lickings.

Producks-That-Wun't-Be: If they find lotsa oil, you mite not see much of yer Carrypoo, yer Canda Geest, yer Perrygreen falkin, yer Hoopingcrain, and yer Mussedcocks.

Mettles: Up till recent, yer fur Northland has bin minin' its own bizness, but now yer whites is comin' in with ther hevvy vestments. Ther startin' to git the lead

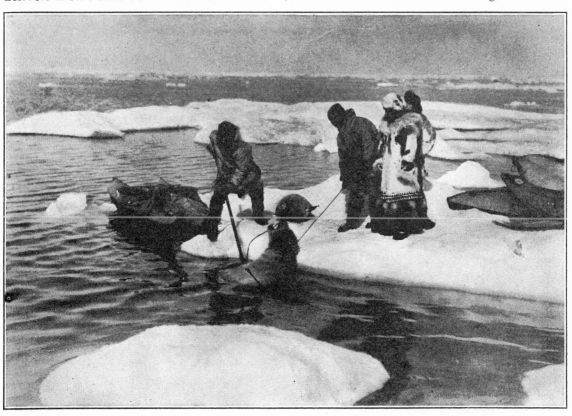

Getting fur cote out of storge

out. There's some gold and a few coppers around yer Grate Slave belt. Also the odd bitta pitchblonde in yer zink...it's pitchblack as a matter of fack and goes to make up yer U-2-3-4.*

Arn ore and other base smettles has bin found on Bafflin Iland and has bin ship'd at mebbe 12 dollar a ton to yer Rear Vallee in Germny. But rolled cold, it's 45 dollar the same ton, so mebbe we shud set up our own guvmit orehouses.

Oyl: Trubble with yer Guvmint, it alwaze works on Commishuns. They 'point a Royl groopie fer to studdy a sertin problim to see what can be done wen it has alreddy bin did by private fellers workin' on strait sallery.

You take yer Nashnul Elergy Bord conducking a Freezability Studdy of yer pipeline wen it's alreddy bin 'ranged fur by Impeerious Oil (wich is reely yer Standerdoyle of New Jerksy). The hole of yer mouth of yer McKinsey's Delter is split up 'tween Golf, Mobeeloyl, Richfeeld, and Shellcans. So wat's the use of granting heerings to Wafflers and Pillution Probers and pertending that they will give out a sertificack of publick conveenients before a penny is dropt?

Yer hole pipeline deepends on who owns the rig, and after we git the shale out, then comes a bigger Shale Out than Hellerween when all that oyl trickles down acrost yer border. Becuz if that linea pipe is gonna cost tenbillyun dollers, we're all gonna have to borry the munny by usin' our Amurrican Xpress Carts.

The Cabnet fella used to be Pastmaster Genrul, Erk Careeruns (that was when Turdo got the Hellyer out of there, too), he sez all we'll git fer leesin' our Articks is a ten pursesent cut of yer Royaltease. Mind ya, that's about as much as yer avrage Rab-eye expecks.

Native Rites: This may jist put the cap on yer untap welth. After all, it's THER native land, and ther startin' to stand on gard fer it agin me and thee.

*CHEERY FEETNOTE: Orville sez it sounds like one of his hyscool yells.

Before the whites got ther eyes on ther land, ther used to be 'bout a hundert thousand Eskamoe. Now there's mebbe 15 thou, thanks to a pox on the white man, both yer small and yer measlies. Most Eskymoes is so sick and tired, they're startin' to stand up fer ther Abridge-in-all Rites.

Lucky fer them, no Eskmoe has ever sined one of them tricker treeties with yer white man. Yer Injian says them treeties ain't worth the paper it's wiped on anyways.** But yer Eskmo is in a better than mishunary posishun, cuz the white man got no rite to grab at his assets.

Yer Minister-of-Northerners-Affairs-that-was (before yer big Cabnet shovel), Gene Cretin, he tried to give conpenstation to yer Native, but that was after them Brother-Hoods in Alasker held up yer Ewe Ass guvmint fer one billyun dollar. Cretin he din't think our Injian Act shud be perform'd that way. But the toon it is a-changing becuz it only takes one native riter fer to cut yer jockular vane of yer pipeline. Mind you, our native fellers is more likely to block the hole thing with a cork injunkshun. I think our Injians 'n Eskmos wanta vote along with yer rast of yer oyl cumpny sockholders. (In case you haven't herd of sich a thing, it's called Demockersee.)

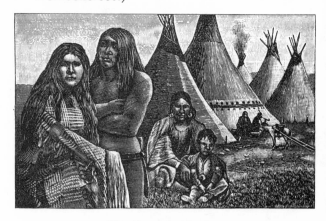

He dimands his rites

**OLD FEETNOTE: Yer Injian first signed up with George yer Third, who at the time was pernounced non mentils in the compost.

U.S. took-over of oil
we hold deer

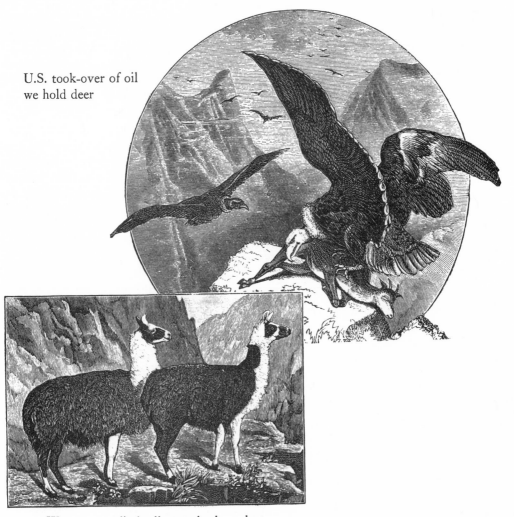

We are poor little llams who have lost

Northwist Passidge: I'm not talkin' bout
yer Spadiner Spressway that was uncovert
some yeers ago. I'm talkin' about yer not-
so-eesy-to-see root that connecks yer A.
and P. Otions.

They bin lookin' fer this ever since
Jack Carter cum thru yer Bill Ile Strait
lookin' fer yer riches of Far Camay. Sir
John F. Ranklin (after him was name yer
Rank Inlet) was sent lookin' fer it . . . and
may still be, becuz he ain't bin herd from
yet. Sam Herney tryed it overland (I shud
say over ice) and went up and out of his
Coppermind. Yer Admirable Parry saled
as far in as yer Melvel Sound . . . yer

Admirable Peery got strait up the Pole,
and Admirable Bird ended up on yer
other Pole.*

It was yer toast of yer Danish, Ronald
Ambudsmen, clames he first done it all
the way with his Scandle Navy Ship
Gjoa. (Sounds Sweetish fer not bein' able
to make up yer mind between Giddap and
Whoa.) In 1940, yer Henry Larseny,
R.C.M.P., got stuck haff way, but finely
got his St. Rock off and circumambulated
the hole root. But ther was a wore on at

*NAVEL FEETNOTE: It's eesy to git confuwsed here.
I ast Orville to repeet all that back, and he said it was yer
Admiral Velvel wat discovered Parry Sound.

the time and nobuddy notissed, exsep mebbe yer Ewe-bote captin lookin' up his peeryscope.

It were 1968 that yer Yanks done it with the biggestanker ever bilt, yer *S.S. Manhatin* (bigger and more expensiv than yer S.S. Kressgee). It wudn'ta made it if yer Canucker ice-broker *Johnnay Macdonald* hadn't pulled a fast one when she seen yer Manhatin-on-the-rocks. They wudda hadda return match strait up in '69, but the game was called by Pee-air Turdo on accounta sovernty.

After yer *Manhatin's* freeassco, they got Bo-ing to desine a plane big enuff to hall six millyun poundsa gas. They cum up with sumthing with a three-wing hellcopper Rotarys. But you'd think with all that gas, they'd go back to yer Dirge-bull like yer Hindyburg er yer Rs-100 fer to git the Hellyum out of there.

Transports: It's hard to find yer way around yer Articks, manely on accounta yer cumpiss don't work that close to yer Norse Pole and ends up giving everybuddy the needle. Sumtimes plains get forcedown, and you mite have to end up eeting nothin' but yer Cannibals soop.

Mane meens of gittin' around is yer Smoemobeel. But last winter a lotta Esks went back to ther dogs when them Arbs got us by the pipeline.

Don't seem to be much place fer yer car on yer tunder. I mind it wen Yellernife had two cars and one trafficking lite. I gess the lite din't work becuz both cars collid with eech other one Sardy nite! (That was before yer Breth-a-liar test.)

Rode bilding is genrully a diaster on accounta yer spring turns yer permyfrost into a quackmire. The one hope seems to be fer yer Ralerode to bind the ties of yer North, but come meltin' time it may turn out to be yer Nashnul Wet Dreem. Most Northerners who wants to git around in yer Artick sircles is jetsettlers. Wunce a yeer, yer suppleye botes brings in rashins of frozen fud. Sounds like shuvellin' cole into Newcassle, er ferlizer back into the barn!

Sitty Life: Agin you'd be s'prised how many natuff peeples has left ther Nomad's Land fer to becum towny foke. Peeple seem to be huddling togither in Greasy Fords, Igluelick, Hey River, Norson Welles, Cake Dorsel, Belly Pay, and Ford Simp's Son.

Yellernite: Hed sitty. Has its own hyrize and a traffick lite wich sez GO all summer. Wich is how this town got its name (peeple stay up all Jooly 'n Awgust). In winters everybuddy gose to bed and fer a change has white nites.

Aklavickle: Town bilt on yer Permerfrost and forced to start its own sinking fund. If that Yellernite hi-rize had bin here, it'd now be a one storee bilding with nine sub-basements. Guvmint bilt a new town on stilts called Inewvic and tried to git Eskmo Resdans to move. But most peefurred to stay where they was, even tho' mosta the old gang tends to disspeer.

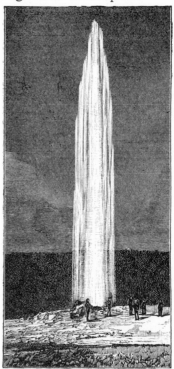

Yeller Nife hi-rise (in winter)

Inewvic: Town holey made by the Federal givmint (sorta like Rockcliff). Has a big round Eskmoe church, St. Igloose, and a licker store that does a millyun dollers a yeer biz. Also its own A and W (cum as you are, but by gosh, stay in yer car), and a furs class hotel. They was gonna call it yer Hilton Stiltin, but a stranger on his way ther ast a native cupple parkad by the rode "How far is yer Eskimo Inn?" and he was tole "None of yer goldurn bizness."

They got TV, thanks to yer Sattiddyite, and Eskmoe kids watch Sezsammy Street like everybuddy elts. (Too bad ther parnts can't git "HeeHar," which is Sezsammy Street fer groan-ups.)

Tuckertoyactup: Yer hindquarters end of yer DUE line (not paid fer yet) on yer Bofors See and manely looked after now by yer Artick chars. This long name meens "the place made cross by a dear." It's a favrit of Toorists becuz you kin buy cheep Injian beeds and Exmo sculpture made in Japanned. It may becum as poplar as Dizzly-land, and is awreddy a kind of Mickey Mouse town.

Alurk: On yer furthist tipoff Ellensmear Iland. Only one furthern North than this is Sandy Claws. No Examoe wud be crazy enuff to live this far North. Animals neether. Nothin' is Alurkin up here but 200 serviceablemen doin' Lord-nose-wat kinda seecret undy-water spearmints.

Rasselewd Bay: Visiters kin get a good taste of mucktuck, wich is yer innards lair of yer sub-cute-tickle of yer ded wale and tastes a bit like them Planterd Peenuts. The game peeple plays up here is good old soft-balls, 'counta it's handy to have a bat in yer hand when them muskeeters comes callin'.

Frozebitcher Bay: Is wher yer effluent sassiety lives . . . rich enuff to have ther own slum. Yer Artick slum is all on the surfiss, incloodin' yer soo-idge.

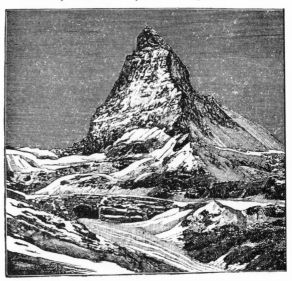

Mountin garbitch, Frozebitcher Bay

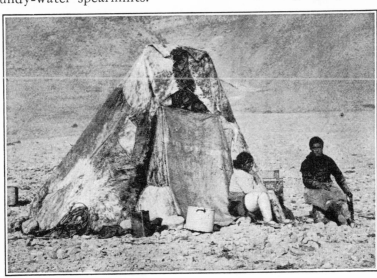

Makin' yer Arctick skin flick

Cheef garbidge cleckter is Ravins, who will eet annything sept Crow. You talk about yer totalled ree-call, that'd be yer Artick garbidge. If you cast yer bred upon them froze waters, it comes back to you next spring in the forma pencil-linen.

This brings up yer Yeckollegy, wich is a envy-ironmintal look at the mess we made. Fer anything we puts on yer perm-frost stays there till yer Last Strump. Nuthin' ever disspeers in yer Artick . . . it's more like yer muther's Attick.

You take TAPS, yer Trans-Alasker Pipe, wich ain't never gonna be bilt. But they got thousands of miles of pipe lion on the ground at yer Prudish Bay jist lion there f'rever. As yer Beerd of Avon sez, "The rust is silents."

Mane consern of us in Canda now is that oyl tankering down yer West Coast from Juno or Pointa Barro. If it gits spilt, that'll be TAPS fer yer B.C. fishy bizness.

* * *

What of yer fewchers? I still think it's yer Artick's tern. As John Deefenbaker sed with his dubble vision, a slummering jiant is waken up. And so's its inhibitants, fer yer Eskamoe don't want to sell his hertage fur a mess of pot. Mind you, they still mite git turned by us into Alkyholicks Unanimuss.

Mebbe the best thing us whites kin do is give the North Waste back to yer Esks, but we better cleer it first with yer Injian and yer Yank. But mebbe by that time the Staits will have bin bot up by yer Arbs, and Canda will be on leash to yer Jap. Then the 49th parrarralell will become yer grate divide between yer Far and yer Middle Eest.

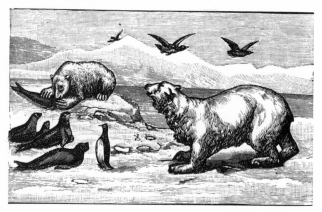

Artick sports — Bares vs. Seals   (in the finals)

Part Three: Yer Rast of Yer Wirld: Ther Parts

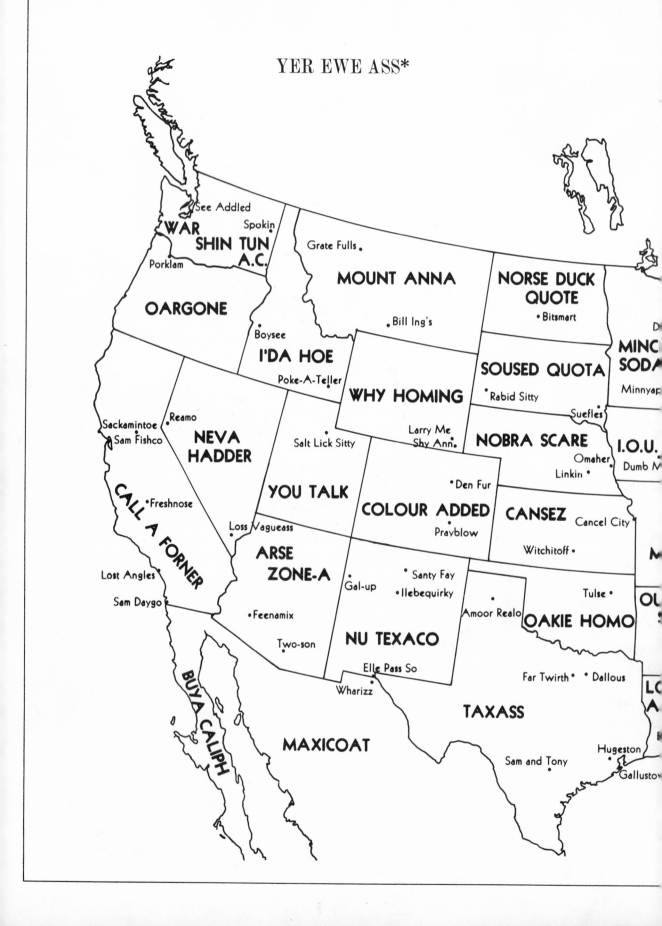

YER EWE ASS*

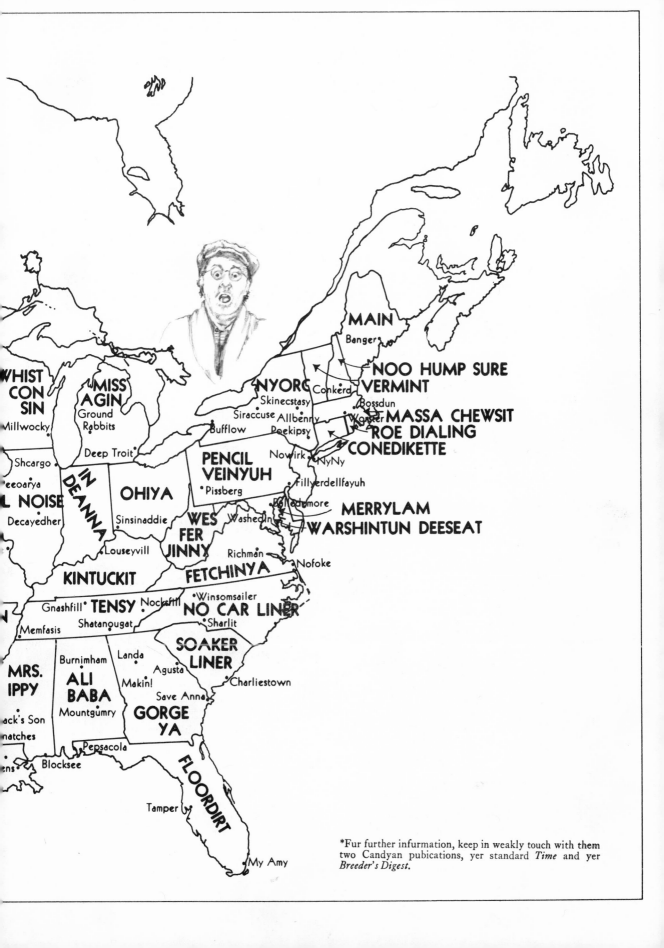

WHIST CON SIN

MISS AGIN
Ground Rabbits

Millwocky

Shcargo

eeoarya

L NOISE

Decayedher

IN DEANNA

OHIYA

Sinsinaddie

Louseyvill

KINTUCKIT

Gnashfill• TENSY

Memfasis

Shatanougat

MRS. IPPY

ack's Son
natches

ALI BABA

Mountgumry

Burnimham

Landa

Makin!

Agusta

Save Anna

GORGE YA

Pepsacola

Blocksee

ens

Tamper

FLOORDIRT

My Amy

Deep Troit

Bufflow

PENCIL VEINYUH

• Pissberg

WES FER JINNY

Washedn

Richman

FETCHINYA

Nockoftll

•Winsomsailer

NO CAR LINER

•Sharlit

SOAKER LINER

Charliestown

Nofoke

MAIN
Bangers

NYORC
Skinecstasy

Siraccuse Allbenny
Poekipsy

Nowirk •NyNy

Conkerd

NOO HUMP SURE
VERMINT

Bossdun

Worster

MASSA CHEWSIT
ROE DIALING
CONEDIKETTE

Fillyerdellfayuh

Balladamore

MERRYLAM
WARSHINTUN DEESEAT

*Fur further infurmation, keep in weakly touch with them
two Candyan pubications, yer standard *Time* and yer
Breeder's Digest.

MEXICO

This place is shape like a big cornycopey-uss, with the big end up yer Staits and the small-bizness end formed into yer penisula of Yuckytan. Ya mite think that was fer to funnul down Ewe Ass ade, but them Mexes shut off the big end 'bout 1924, so that yer Yank took-over never got a chants to took. Them "dum pee-ons" still owns 55% of themselves.

The one reel dum thing they do is yer Bull-fit. And they do it evry week in Urenas all over, like at Teeheewanna, Acapella, and Mexcosity. (I think yer swift Canadyans at Canneda Packers gits better wurk done.) They got this fella, yer Tory-adore, who's a regular Mexcun yumpin' bean, and they git him to wave his red undyware rite under yer cosy nostrils of a big Black Angers. And this is after that aminal has alreddy bin stuck with a

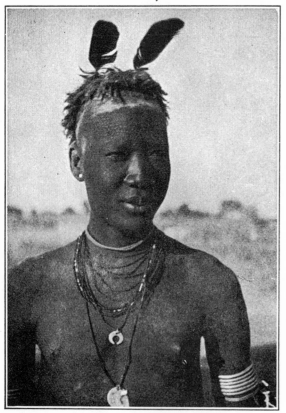

Mickey Mouse bullfitter

buncha tooth-picks, what they call yer peckerdillos.

There stands the Tory-adore in his light soot and Mickey Mouse club hat, waitin' fer the bullrushes. Sumtimes he gits impale by one of the big horny devils till he looks like a Marciano cherry. That's because the dern fool turns his back on yer bull-rush and jist asts fer this rip-snorter to give it to him up the backside. (That's what these Ringos call yer "momentuss trooth." I think the trooth is he shud hi-tail it over behind that peenalyty box they have at the side.) Now I know yer Black Angers and I've took a lot from t'other end. But I prefur to spred that than to git *myself* spred fur and wide.

Mind you, it's yer bull wat gits it in the end, fer these fits is all fixed. I never herd of a bull gittin' two eers and a peece a tale from a Matted-door. (That's the fella delivers yer "cooze de grass.") And everybuddy throws ther hat in the ring like Deefenbaker at a convenshun, and nobuddy thinks to call yer S. Peace of A.

SENTER AMURKA

Bertish Houndyerass: It's south of the boarder down Mexco's way. It's noan to most Canadyans as the place where Pee-air Truedough gose skinny dipping with his snorker.

Wotamalla, Nickeraqua, Hi Costa Reeka, Else Alvadoor, and yer Bananama Zone: Is yer belt fer yer United Froots Bunch to hang onto. But yer Gay Libation made them change ther name to "United Brands." But that don't go more'n skin deep with yer banana Republickan biznessmen.

WEST UNDYS

Cuber: Got Castroed fifteen year ago and not much bin herd from sints, sept wen they wanted to buy tranes from us. And our lanlord, yer Ewe Ass, suspeckted our loco-motivayshuns.

Jamaker: Has mostly moved to Tronta, wher they give a Sandy Claws prade in the middle a summer, oney better. It's jist after us Ornjmin has tootled our floots, but these fine-fetherd Carnal-rama fellas with ther loose limbos sure make us look pale in every way.

Hatey: Was under yer Tomtom Mycoots (the local Gestapoo with sun glasses), but now they is welcummin' tooriests agin . . . and thinkin' of changin' ther place's name to LOVEY.

Dominicancan Repubic (Captol: Sen Dagringo): Has not yet got over Prez Linen Johnson's saving them in '68, wen yer Murines landed and got yer sityation well out of hand.

Trimdad and Tobasco: The only place Canda has ever bin accused of Imperiousism . . . and yer lokal Royl Bank got the drafts in ther winders to prove it.

Barbydose: One of yer lesser Aunt Tilly's and full of as many Canucks down there as we got Barbydolls and Trimdaddyos up here.

Yer Grand Bananas: Anuther buncha chartered Canadyans infesting an Iland fer seven days and tryna pertend they live like Eepee Tailor and Casey Irving, who do this kinda thing permanint and tacks free.

Barenuda: Not one Iland like I thot, but a hole buncha them, both yer longs and yer shorts. They is sed to be yer furthest north corl groop.* Biggest imports: by-sickles and hunnymooners.

SOUSE AMURKA

Sum say this place is a dagger pointed rite at the hart of yer Ant's Articka. So them poor Pengwins is jist sittin' ducks. But that's the way yer Staits seeze S. Amerkens. In Canda, we mange to eggnoar the fack that the hole continence exists.

Venusazalea: Captoll sitty: CRACKERS. This used to be one of yer havesnot nay-shuns. But they got well oiled last yeer and started givin' us the runs fer our munny.

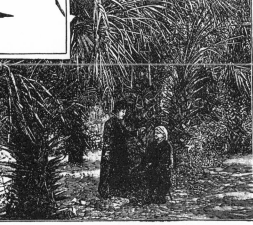

Yer nashnul realitty

Yer nashnul dreem

*REEFOOTNOTE: The wife says her Parry Sound Sintennial Quire is yer more northern corl grupe. Biggest, too. They have a corus of over 60, sept the wife, who's 58.

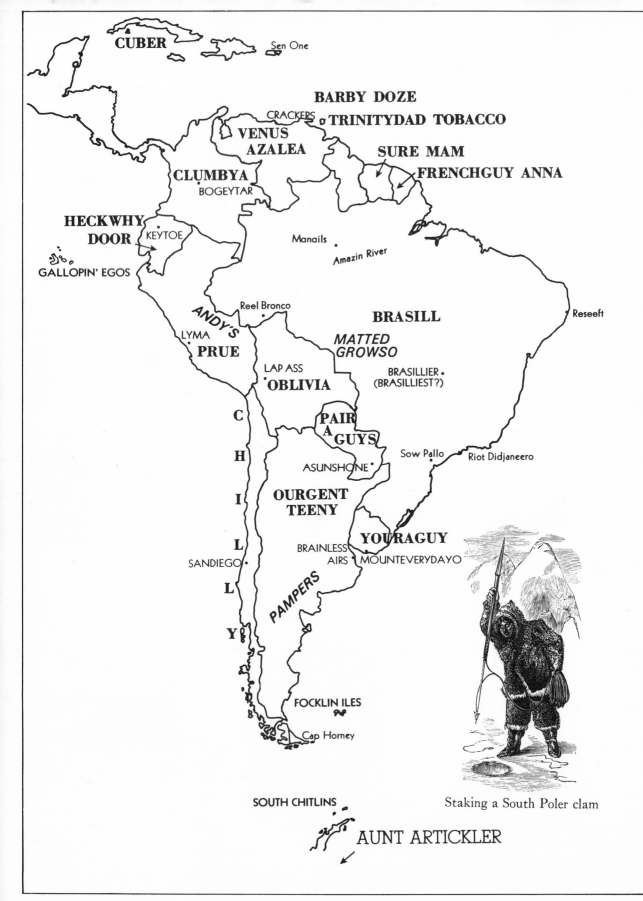

CUBER

Sen One

BARBY DOZE

CRACKERS ▫ TRINITYDAD TOBACCO

VENUS AZALEA

SURE MAM

FRENCHGUY ANNA

CLUMBYA

BOGEYTAR

HECKWHY DOOR

KEYTOE

Manails

Amazin River

GALLOPIN' EGOS

ANDY'S PRUE

Reel Bronco

BRASILL

Reseeft

LYMA

MATTED GROWSO

LAP ASS

OBLIVIA

BRASILLIER (BRASILLIEST?)

C

PAIR A GUYS

H

Sow Pallo

Riot Didjaneero

I

ASUNSHONE

L

OURGENT TEENY

YOURAGUY

BRAINLESS AIRS

MOUNTEVERYDAYO

L

SANDIEGO

PAMPERS

Y

FOCKLIN ILES

Cap Horney

Staking a South Poler clam

SOUTH CHITLINS

AUNT ARTICKLER

Senter Amurka, West Undys, and Souse Amurka

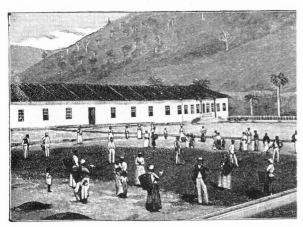

Cawfee — the daily grind

Clumbya: Cappittall: BOGEYTAR. Perdooces much of yer world's coffy, so is listed as a has-bean country. Everyone lives hy here on accounta yer Andy, the world's longest mountain chain . . . and so far nobuddy's pulled it.

Extrador: Captall: KIDDO. Follers the genral rool of most Souse Merken countrys by bein' rooled by a Genral.

Prue: Cappittal: LYMA. Also has-beans. It had more wen yer Inkys was in charge, but yer Spanish Fly-be-nite Conkistyerdoors under yer PeerzArrow fixed them in no-time flat. Monty Zoomer's revenge was to name Lake Titty-ka-ka in his mammery.

Prue is yer except to the Genral Rool and is even flurting at this moment with yer Universal Frencheyes.

Oblivia: Captill: LAP ASS. Has a left genral fer a change. But he got overooled and left at the invite of yer Merken ambassy, who figgered a better blow fer demockersee wud be yer far rite rather than yer outside left.

Chilly: Cap: SAN DIEGO. Is co-opulating with the new U.S. polissy of not interfeering with yer avrage right-winger Dick Tater, now that yer preevious encumbrance has come to a brupt and fine-All-Endy.

Pairaguy: Captall: ASUNSHONE. This place hasn't perduced much . . . some wild roomers and a cuppla bony-fried Natzys.

Youraguy: Captull: MONTY'S VIDEO. Way ahed of the rast of the world. Had galuping inflayshun back in 1950 and bankrupcherd itself. Has deesided to fite it out on the beeches and go toorist. Watch for the Biznessman's Speshul, wich is holding bank presdents fur ransom by yer Toopy-Marrows, the lokal tarewrists.

Urgenteeny: Cap: BONUS AIRS. The biggest beefer of them all, thanks to yer grouchos. Now led by yung lady presdent, who has jist took over her husbins (One Prone) posishun.

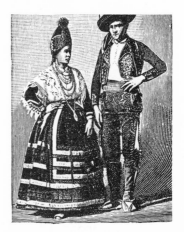

Groucho and frend

Bra Sill: Almost as big as yer Ewe Ass and with an ever bigger mouth (Amazin), wich emptees reglar. Us Canucks is down ther sittin on our Brasscans.

Cap: Reel Dingy Nero. No, by gol, Bra Sillier! They folk moved ther captall outa range of yer Action like we dun with Ottawa in Bytown daze.

Yer Guyanus: Yer Birtish, yer French, and yer Dutch (Surema'am). A jungel under three flags.

Yer Cake a Gud Horn: Sits rite on the enda yer Chilly tip. It's a big senter fer wind-gatherin' and a well-noan ship disturber.

Yer Focklin Ilands: Jist a dip to the rite of yer Horn. B'longs to yer Queen Liz (the sovern, not the bote, which is now a botel offa Callfornia and takes in roomers).

Ya'll never bleeve this, but the inhibitants is a mixed batch of Scotsmen and sheep, jist like yer John-a-Goats!

AN TARTKICKER

Capital place: Wherever yer King Pengwin happens to hunker down. If youse ever want to go south fer the winter, this is the most south place that has the most winter. It's colder than an instinkt reeplay of a fifty-first weddin' annaversery.

It perdooces 90 pissent of yer wirld's ice (no mix), and sum Callfornia ticoon is alreddy thinkin' of towin' iceburgers up his way and sellin' 'em retale after he's nocked ther blocks off.

Mebbe there's no bizness like snow bizness. Everybuddy is startin' to git a cold toe-hold on yer Antartickler ice shelf, incloodin' yer Jap and yer Roosian . . . mebbe on accounta yer Jap has Tuna'd out most of yer Specifick Ocean, and yer Serviets has bin trawlin' around doin' the same thing by Cod.

One of yer nooest soreses of proteen is a little shrimpy invertineebriate called yer Krill, and there's billyuns, trillyuns, probly krillyuns of 'em down there. So you jist watch these two pree-daters, yer Jap and yer Roosian, move in fer the Krill.

YER ANTIPPYDEEDOODAHS

Oztrailyuh: Cap: CANTBEARHER. Always wanted to go down under and see great Quantustees of Cola bares in yer Youclipptus trees, er them Kangyruse

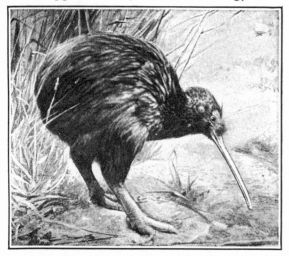

Kee-wee drinkin' shoo polish

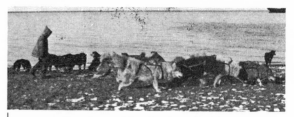

Byrd watching in Ant Artkicker

boxin' and playin' tennace. (They even have speshul Kangroo corts.)

And they sure got some queer birds out there in yer BackOut . . . Keewees, Buck Dilled Flatterpusses, and a Cockertwo. But the one I'd like to see is the burd sticks his hed in the ground and thinks you can't see him, jist like yer avrage Water-gaiters. We have relations down under, and one of them sent us a Osterrich aig fer Chrissmuss. The darn thing was sich a size the wife din't have a pan big enuff in the kitch'n, so I biled the aig in the bath-tub. Jist as well I did, fer it was the only room in the house had an aig-cup big enuff.

Task-mania: I thot it sounded like the wife during spring cleenin', but turns out to be a nyland offa the sow-eest shore of yer Come-on-Welth. It used to be called Van Demon's land, but the name got changed by them clever little Taskmanian devils.

Newzie Land: Cap: WULLINGTUN. Don't have yer topical climutt, but is more meen-tempert like ours. Sept, like Oztraileyer, it's yer arsey-versey. They're puttin' on Noxenema when we're gittin' into our ballbrigands.

Ya'd think it was olde Ingaland or Victororia, B.B.C., if it wasn't fer them Marys. Yer Mary is yer ridge-in-all settler come from yer micro-Polly-neezys from yer Cooked Ilands and yer Rarertungers. Seems they used to eat "long pig," wich is meerly p'lite talk fer cannonballism. But that's obscolene now, so "long pig no see."

Newzies used to be under th'inflooence of yer Grater Britons. But since they subscried to yer C'lumbo Plan, they now git Amurrican TV shows like Peeter Focks.

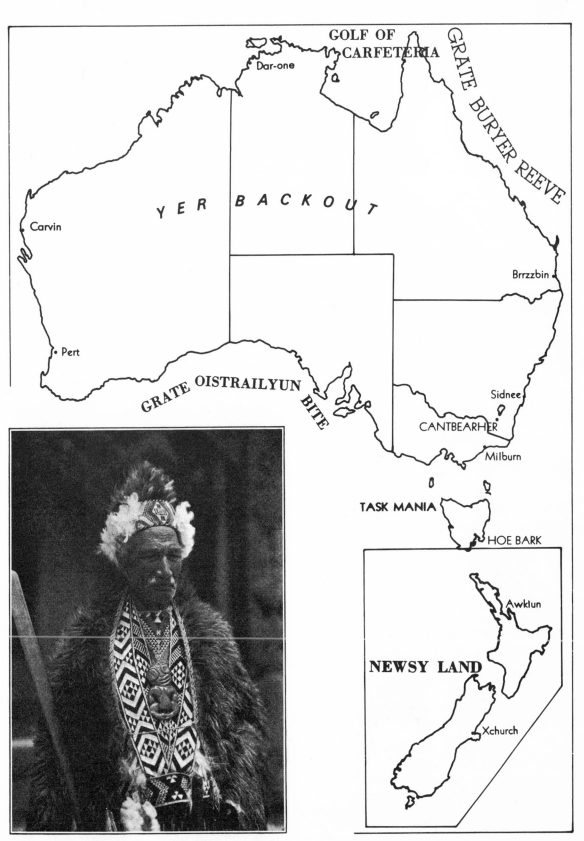

GOLF OF
CARFETERIA

GRATE BURYER REEVE

Dar-one

Y E R   B A C K O U T

Carvin

Brrzzbin

Pert

GRATE OISTRAILYUN BITE

Sidnee

CANTBEARHER

Milburn

TASK MANIA

HOE BARK

Awklun

NEWSY LAND

Xchurch

Mary with Eester hat

Yer Antippydeedoodahs

YERP

Strickly speekin', yer continence shud be circumsized by a large body with water in it. But you take North Amurka 'fore they druv a canal thru yer Pissmus of Anima, er Affker 'fore they drejjed up yer Sue-us. So let's not be two picky-une* (as the gittarrh player sed) and inclood Yerp.

Grate Britten: Cappitall: LENNON. This arraignmint of Kelts, Gales, and Angled Sacksons is reely a continence all by itself, even tho' it's in yer Common Markup. It's still hard fer me to think of peeple that speek Anglish as Yerpeens, becuz you take yer Yerpeen, ther mostly forners.**

Anglin: The news from Dredneedle Street is gittin' worst, so I gess the best export they got these daze is yer Royl Family. They bin sending them all on toor reglar like yer "Stoodent Prints."

After wat we've seen lately from yer 'lected repreehensitives, I think yer Kings and Kweens aren't so irreverent and immateeriel after all. They haven't had one of ther bunch unpeeched since Charley First was impared by that Crum Well.

*FINGERNOTE: The wife don't think I shud use words like that wen I dunno wat they reely meens. She sez it to Orville wen he's doin' sumthin' he shoodn't with his nose.

**FURRIN FEETNOTE: Oney thing forn about yer Anglish is that they drive on the Gee! side instedda the Haw!

I like that bunch from yer House at Wincer becuz they're country folks. They don't hang around yer Buckinghams Palissaid all the time. As soon as they c'lect ther Royaltees, they're off up to yer Ballmorals, growsing (shooting peasant), er taking a tramp over to yer Moores. They kin deel with all classes without puttin' on side. Why lookit the fellas they married . . . that Greek sailer, yer Prints Reegional, and the Brownie-snapper Tony Strongarm Jones.

Meself, I'm parshul to that Princess Anne of Green Stables, who had the dubble weddin' last yeer along with Stumpy Tom Cobley on yer Munchin' Date with Elmwood Clover.

Scotsland: It's like the barnyard . . . gotta be careful how I step. Fer the wife's side of the family was mostly displased Glass-Weejuns who got pulled up from ther roots in the Goreballs and have bin short a few heirs ever since.

We in Canda has got a langridge problem. But it's not from yer French becuz most all of them speeks Anglish. (Mind you, they only do it wen one of us trys to speek the French first.) But it's yer Scot that can't seem to git the hang of it. I've known Mcs and Macs bin heer fur forty yeer, and the need for sub-tittles gits worse. They must meet in seecrit every

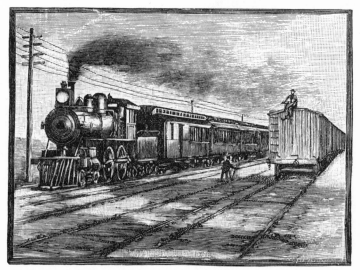

How yer Scotsman Flys

week and practiss to see wich one can speek the most broken Canadyun. That's why they still sound like them Tattood Edinburgers what come over to skirl ther kilts fer us Canadyan Nashunal Inhibishunists.

Wails: That's wat it's called, but I call it Singin' and a sound fer sore eers wen all them Welchers gits together and has a sing-song . . . wat they call a Studfod. The wife she even likes that bumpy grinder "Tom Jones", altho' meself I didn't care too much fer him in that moovy with everyone sloppin' ther fud.

IRAland: Wen I was yung, biggest day of the yeer wud be yer gloryass twelfa Joo-lye. There'd be floot-tootlin' and drum-stickin', and us boys wearin' our Ornj sashays and them pill-box hats jist fer to make them Cathlicks mad.

But I don't go no more fer to see King Belly on his Whitehoarse. Over in Ulcer, they still have the Ornj crushes, and they have a ring-tailed snorter of a bang-up time burnin' ther busses and britches behind them. Wen it comes to the point where baby-carridges is havin' a neer-miss from yer home-made bomms, then it's time to stop fightin' about wich Sundy scool you went to. Seems to me yer nashnal Antrim these days is "If yer Irish, come into the Funeral Parler."

Yer Chanel Eyelands: Home of Five poor-fumes . . . Jerzy, Gurney, Alternitnee, and Stark . . . but I think the Number 5, Evenin' in Pars, is made neer Brantfurd.

Anyways, they all speek the French but b'long to Britten, so they're way ahed of us with yer Bilge 22.

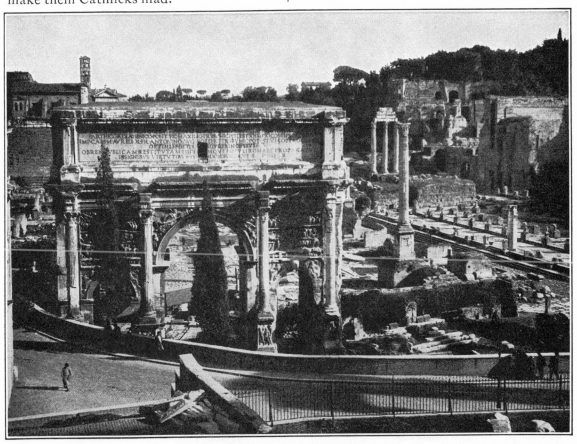

St. Pall's after yer Berlitz

Fran's: Capitol: PARS. Apart from kissin' Arb's barenooses last winter, Fran's has bin quiet lately, giver take th'odd Atomickal boom as they passed ther Newcleer tests over yer Murderoe Athole. Mosta yer fall-off cum over Newzieland. Only thing Canadyan got infected was yer skipper of yer *Greenpeas*. Yer French Murines was as good as ther word when they sed they'd keep an eye out fer him.

But that new Premiere, Valerie Discard Disdain, won't let any more bums off. Takes a woman to bring back common cents.

Spane: Captoll: MADRIB. Still fightin' that Sivvil Servants War they had in '36-'39. The trubblemakers is now them Loylist Baskerds who are holed up in yer Pairnees and got no place to go but down. That's what happens when you put all yer Basks in one exit.

Porchgull: Capitul: LISPIN. Used to take dick-tation, but reecently threw up and got demockersy. Now they're plannin' on givin' it to ther Affercans possessed in Hangcola and Moe Sam's Beak.

Jibhalter: Spainyards keep trying to git Britons offs that rock jist this side of ther Casteel slope, but them Prude-dental Insurients keeps tellin' 'em to stay put.

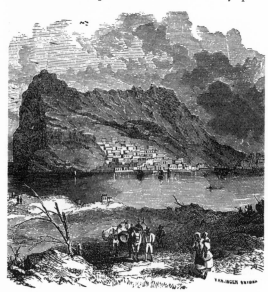

Yer jib rock

Popillation is split between Bertish offishuldums and yer Barbie apes.

Malted: A small base plase that yer Bertish uses as a airport when the lokels aren't tarin' a strip offa them. Yer Birtish lyon is trying offal hard not to make yer Maltese cross.

Ittly: Caputol: ROAM. Is rumored to be goin' out of bizness and jist about to git the boot. There'll be a "Everything Must Go" sail, and they'll all take yer Leonardo Dubinsky and imgrate acrost to yer Westend of Tronto, where they all has reelations. If you don't b'leeve Rome wasn't bilt in a day in sluburban Hogtown, jist ask Daisy Lewis.

Billy Davis started his next 'lection campaign in the Vatican-can. He had a noddience with yer Pope. (You'd wonder where they'd git a noddience fer a thing like that.) Fer you take Billy Davis, he'd be mebbe Angle-can and you take yer avrage Pope, he'd be Roamin Cathlick. And they're even goin' to name a street after Billy there. Madgin' seein' a street in Nables called yer Via Davisbill.

Monicker: A small prince'spaltitty on yer Coat Dasewer above yer Nees. Its mane bizness is spinning weels and braking banks at Monty's Carload. Hedman is Prince Raindeer, who is very devote and insists on Grace before eech meel.

Swishland: Cappital: BURN. Looks like a buncha mountins with sum bilt-in tax shelters. But here's a country speeks three differnt langridges, and nobuddy has fit with eech other fer hunderds of yeers. They started yer Red Crotch fer everybuddy elts!

Never mind yer by-lingams . . . er even yer yoony-. Let's encurge all that malty-culchure and have lotsa offishul langridges, startin' with Eyetalian, Euchre-anium, Japanee, and Low Scotch. Let's hear it fer yer three-way Swish!

Lux'emburg: Cap: ditto. The place that makes sope used by nine out of ten screened stars. They also make munny out of importing Merrican cars . . . I think that's what "Tax Dodges" meens.

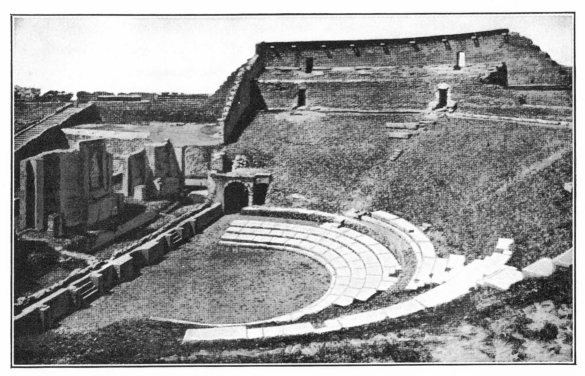

Roman Quorum after Whirld Cup Final

Bellygum: Captl: BRUSTLES. Th'oppsit of Swishland and more like us. Everybuddy here is a seprater, both yer Flemmer and yer Wall-loon, and they're at each other like nives all the time. (Mebbe they're mad cuz they don't run that Congo line no more.) Ther King looks like a nice one, even tho' they call him Bad-one.

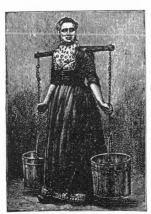

Bulgin girl with big cans

Haulend: Cap: THE HAIG. Any Canajyan serviceableman who was overseezed got a warm cockel in his hart for this place, even tho' we had a ruff time in yer Shelled Eskyouwary with them Pansy Divishuns. Since the war, a lotta Dutch has come over here. That's oney fare, because a lotta Canadyans got in Dutch and brung them out here fur to settle gradjally in yer (Hollander) Marshes.

Demark: Cap: COPE'N HANG'EM. I 'gree with that song "There's nuthin' like a Dane." Copinghaven is the smileyest town I ever seen, and I don't jist meen yer Frivolee Garden. Yer Son don't shine much, but the peeples faces do.

They got a clime-mutt makes Killerloo seem like Myammy. Mind you, that raw eest wind is good fer yer butterfatcontent, and they must make quite a poultry sum on ther aigs. Must be the best place in the wirld fer to be a small farmer . . . and I feel I'm gittin' shorter every yeer. Wonder if that cheery-beery Carl Holeman wud trade places?

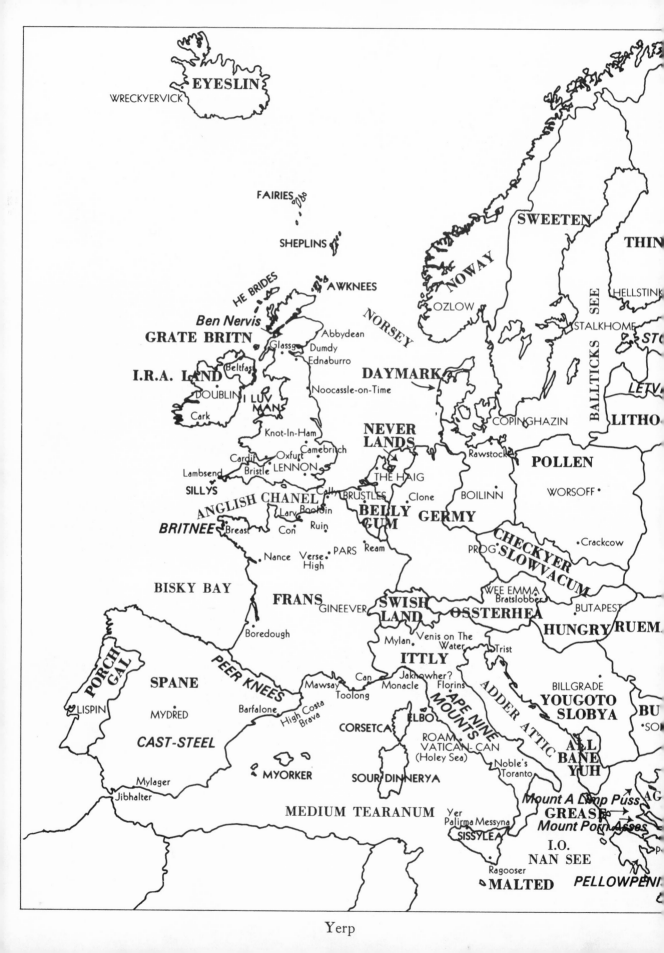

Yerp

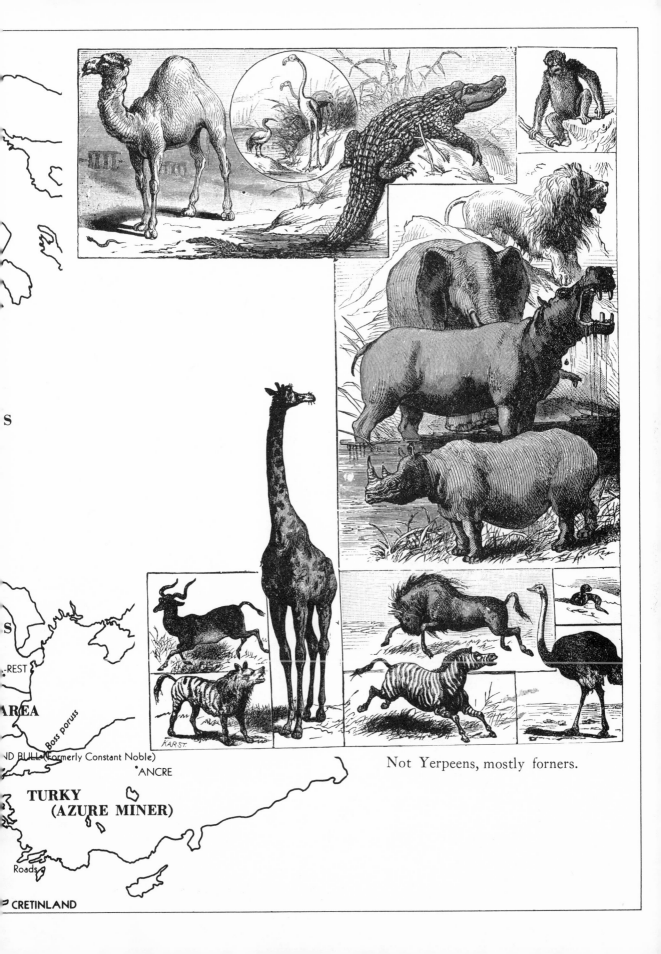

Not Yerpeens, mostly forners.

S

S

REST

AREA

Boss poruss

ND BULLA (Formerly Constant Noble)

ANCRE

**TURKY
(AZURE MINER)**

Roads

CRETINLAND

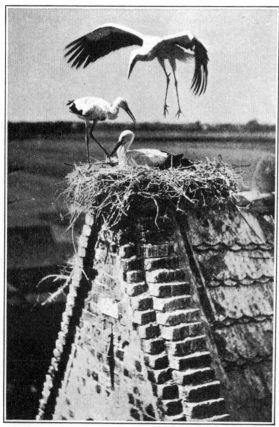

Stork Club (Hamstersdam)

Icyland: Cap: RICKYERVICK. Last yeer one of ther ilands made an ash of itself, and now peeple is livin' offa the new larva. They got a Common House 800 yeer older'n anybuddy's. I gess freedom keeps better on ice. Don't make a lotta noise about it anyways. Ever heer an Icelander talk? . . . jist as soft as two old mades whisprin' in cherch.

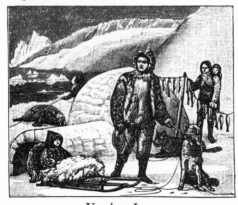

Yer last Lapp

Noway: Cap: BIRKIN. A lot like Muskoker when you watch the Fjords go by. Sounds even more like home when you lern only 4 purrsent of land is fit fur farmin'. Nice down-home, down-t'urth peeple. (Or shud I say down-to-rock?) Still, they make a good livin' cuttin' firs fer to make noospapers and charging all them trolls on yer hyways.

Sweeten: Cap: STUCKHOME. Is as cold as Noway is wet. But they sure know how to stock homes with a fine croppa high-steppin' blonde bangtails. The wife wants to noe how I noe sich a thing. I told her I seen it fer myself in that maggazeen our boy bot that makes you hold yer breth . . . *Panthouse.*

Finishland: Cap: HELLSTINKY. Must be the fastest foke in the wirld, give or take a few Lapps. J'ever see them run out of a sawnoff bath, make angels in the snow, and run back in before they was blew perminently? But yer Fin can stand bein' in heat er cold till Helsinky's over.

Letvia, Stoneya, and Litho-anyus: Three diffrent names fer one Pete-bog. Yer Lithos has got the oldest living tungs in Yerp, and, b'leeve me, they use them agin ther Roosian masterds every chance they git. Yer Letts mostly live in ther capitall, Riggle, and refoose to speek the Roosian, but take a leef from ther own book writ in Lettish. Yer Stoneyuns give us them gorjuss blonde girl exorcists with the big red balls over ther heds.

Germny: Is divide into yer Eest and yer Wast, jist like us in our Gray Cups. Yer Eest is yer Commonest part. They walled therselves off from the Wast when they all got to the Berling point. Having bifurk-dictated therselfs like that, they don't do much trade with yer Common terns.

Yer Wast Germns is much more export at sending produks our way, sich as Folk'swagons, Hamburg, Clone, and Bonnbonns.

Po-land: Cap: WARSORE. Yer Pole is like us Irish . . . willin' to die fer his country in a forn feeled, but be gol-derned if he'll ever work in it wen he's there. But dum? Fergit all them polished jokes. The capitall, Worsoff, is a regular hothouse of branes. It's got more PhDs per square hed than yer Hot House Univursty of Tronto.

Checkyerslowbackinya: Cap: PROG. The word "Prog" don't sound like much, but I bet it's the prittiest sitty ther is, incloodin' Pars with its Iffy Tower. After 1968, we got a lotta Checks in Canda . . . and not one turnd out to be a blank.

Hungry: Cap: BUDDYPEST. Wenever two or three of thim are gather together, then ya got two or three p'litickal partees. Ther wimmen cud give others lessons on th'art of bein' femminim. I wish the men wud jist stop argyin', shuddup, and lissen.

Ossterrhea: Cap: WEE EMMA. Got over bein' power-Hungry 50 yeer ago. Now takes it eesy beetin' ther harts in three quarters the time as they sit on yer sidewocks with a cuppa coffee . . . and a dish at the side fer the creem.

Yugo-ta-slobber-ya: Cap: BILLGRAD. Was foundered out of yer first World War after yer Leega Nayshuns give up tryna seprate yer Slobs from yer Croats. It's now s'posed to be a hard Red state, but you can still wonder round everywhere free . . . and mebbe even git a chants to see Tito thru the tulips.

Remainya: Cap: BUCK-A-REST. Never mind all this talk about steelin' aigs as the first step in a Reminyin resspy. These fellers has stole ther own country back from the Serviet . . . wich is more than we dun so far with yer U.S.

Bulge-area: Cap: SOFEEYA. I hear ther still on the party line.

All-brane-yuh: This has got to be one of yer leest-noan lands on urth, 'spite the fack that the captall sitty is the same as mine: TIRANA! All braneyuns don't seem to git along with nobuddy but yer Red Chinymen, who supplize them with enuff starch to keep up ther second front.

Grease: Cap: ATHN. This kernel of Westerned demockersey has now give up its kernels and brung back sivilianization. Nice to have the home of Sockertease and Arstoddle back in the foaled. Mebbe they'll send our Tronto Aggernuts the Golden Fleas to git into ther pants and make them move tords yer Graycup.

Creet: Cap: CANNYER. The place that most peeple dig. Archeeolljists have bin hangin' around Nossus to find out how they bilt a sibileyezation based on Bull. What makes them ex-Creetins any differnt from us?

YER AZURE MINERS

This part don't fit into yer avrage continence. Mebbe that's why it gives us so much trubble, always putting its square peg into our round hole.

Turky: Cap: ISTANDBULL, farmerly Constantnoble. Used to sit on its Ottoman and gobble up its naybors. But thim Turkeys bin pritty quiet fer decayeds till them Geek huntas tryed to pull off yer cooze-day-tat on yer Iland of Sidepress . . . and that brung yer Turky outa the straw. He moved in, preepaired to stay, jist like yer mother-in-law.

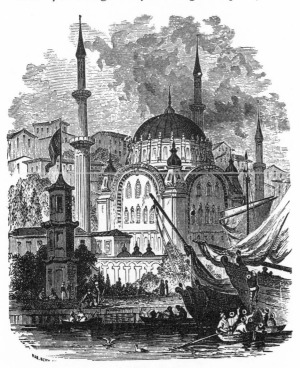

Holday Inn, Athns

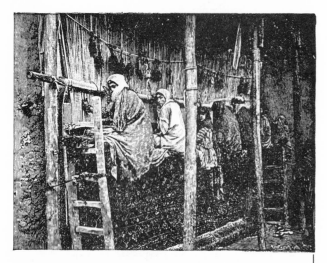

Hardy wallhangers git weavin' in Standbull

Cheef export seems to be that opee-ate of the peeple, Hero-win, but yer Turk dismisses this ugly roomer as so much poppy-crop.

Sidepress: Cap: NICK'LLSEEYA. This ile was run by yer Orthoduck Archy Bishop Vycarious wen yer Greek kernels made ther moovemint tords Eno-sis, wich is not yer frooty salts but the amanglemation with yer Greasin' manelined acros̓t yer I-own-one See. They were hopin' to cook yer Turky's goose before they had time to git across yer Bossforce and land on Farmergooseter.

It was our boys under yer Untied Nation Secyurity blankets got cot in the middle. Us Canadyins is 'sposed to act as a bufferin state, but turns out *we* git the hedake.

Don't see how ther cudha bin any confoozion about the uniforms. Yer Turks have them harum-scarum pants and curled up slippers and hats like Shriners. Them Greaks has big tassholes on ther hats, pompoms on ther shoes, and them little Nashnul Belly dancer skirts that'd put the wind up anybody. And in the middle was our fellas swettin' it out in that Eunuchfication uniform, the one that makes them look like yer green hornet that gives out the parking tickets.

YER MIDLEAST

Seeriac: Fifteen hundert yeer ago, ther captoll, Damasskiss, was yer senter of the wirld. I s'pose that's why ther Goalan life is to reech them Hites agin.

Lesbynon: Sentered on yer Bayroutes. Has a by-thingamul rangemint with a Cristyun presdent and a Mussle-im Prime-minister. Wud like to be the Riveera of yer Midleest, but is becoming better noan as a harbor for All Fattah gorillas.

Earack: Cap: BAGGYDADS. Is where we all got started, fer yer Garden of Eatin was down at the Junkshun of yer Tigerrs and Fraidies Rivers. It's not what it was, sints it's now called Shatt All Arb (look it up if you don't b'leeve me).

It still supplize most of the world with dates (sept on Sardy nites). It's also well-oiled, 'speshully since last year, wen we all started payin' inter-nasally.

They've had ther sepertists trubbles, too. A packa wild Kurds has bin hard to subdude, but yer mane guvmint finely come to turms with them, jist so yer Kurds woodn't git in the whay.

Jordon: Captall: AHMAN! Famuss fer its Ontaryo whines.

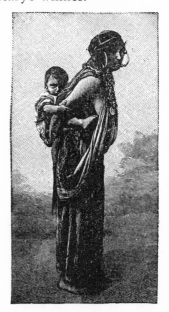

Arb Bed-one

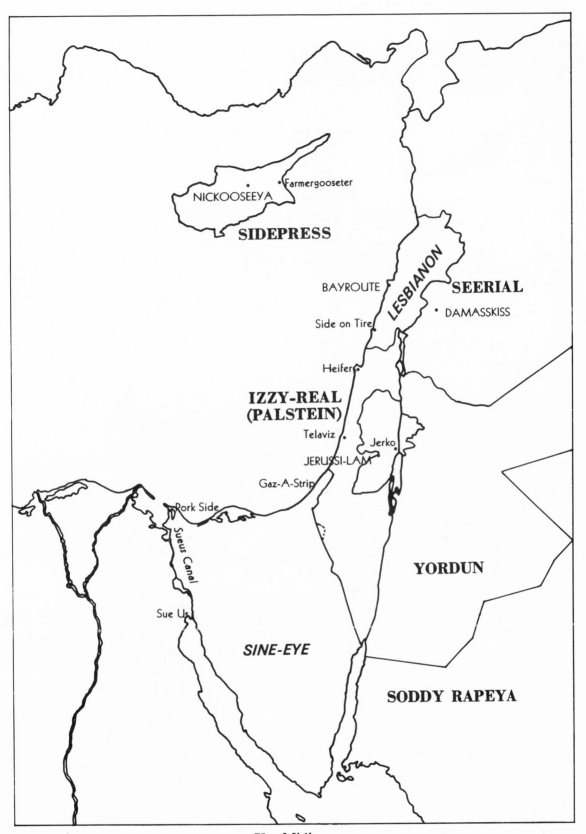

Yer Midleast

Oman: Pritty barn and named after that bird wat spilt his seed on the ground. Muscat, the cappittall, is the home of nomads who love to Rambel.

Yehmen: Dunno what it's in Aden of. Sounds like the cry of yer Gay Livers.

Shoddy Arapeyuh: Capitall: UNLIMITED. The hart of the Arb wirld, where Sheeks are a dollar a dozen.

Izzy-reel: Was the name give to Jake the Smooth, brother of Hairy Heehaw, after he rassled with The Angel (a Sweetish rassler). And them Izzy-realittes has bin rasslin' fer a place to stay ever sints.

These peeple started out as farmers, went into bizness, but went back to the farm as kibbitzers. That don't meen lookin' over someone elt'ses shoulder, but putting it to the weel along with everybuddy else.

Yer Issraley is yer pie-in-ear, doin' everythin' our incesters done a hundert yeer ago . . . and sirrounded on all sides by ther own kinda whoopin' Injians.

Now yer Izz-rale is not the same as yer Palestine. It's eazy to git mixed up, 'speshully if you reeds yer Bibel. Yer Palestinninans was the ones uprooted purt neer thirty yeer ago and has ever sints bin livin' in Nomad's Land. And now they're so darn desprit, they'd like the rest of us fer to try livin' in the same place. If a man lives in terror, don't take much fer to make him a terrorwrist. Even a groundhog has to have his own hole to crawl intuh.

Ther seems to be a new spurt among the yung Izz-reals fer to dò somethin' about this. Hope so before yer next Olymphic game, becuz men without a country to root fer makes bad sports.

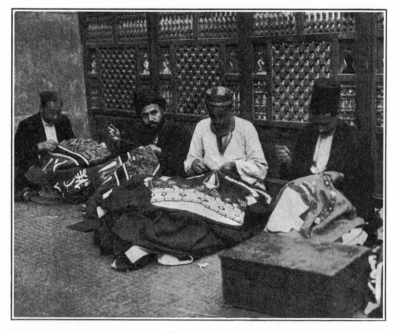

Bizarr men

YER AZURE

Serviet Roosia: (Das Kapital: MA'S COW.) Foundered by Trotsy and Lemin and give over to yer Stallion, hoo past it on to Kruschen with a dose of Salts.*

Anybuddy who has crost it will reelize why it's called yer Reel Muther. To go from one side to t'other, from Lemongrad to Flathosstock, is like transgressin' haffa yer urth ... 'speshully takin' all them stepps to go in and out of yer Urnals. They even got sum salty seeze, like yer Arl and yer Castrian, in the middle of ther big planes. And some long drinksa water of rivers, yer big broaD Nipper, and yer even bigger Vulger. And one bobby doozer of a volleyuminus lake, Buckall. Pluss they got yer most friggid part of the wirld ... wirst than our own Articks ... yer Sighbeerier.

When it comes to them seeze at ther northern end parts, they freeze sollid, both yer Bare-Ends and yer Ballticks. It's only in summer that mosta yer sturrgeons will come up stream to make caffy-are.

Alla yer farmers is well-eddicated, most of them Stalingrads from yer KeyF U., er yer Smollensk Tech. And yer Uke-rain is s'posed to be the oldest grannry in the wirld. But collidge farmers can't make water and they can't git the hail out of the way neether. So the last few yeers they

*DISARMING FEETNOTE: So far, a lotta tock and no ackshun.

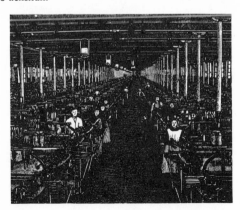

Vodky brake

bin importin' our granes ... and we bin importin' ther belly dancers and hockey players. D'you mind that Bullshy fella Mickey Britchnyripoff? He's now doin' a pass d'un fer our Belly peeple, and they're even writin' a hole corpse de danse fer him called "Lay Siphleeds." (You'd wunder why they'd wanta do a one-two-three kick about yer sociable diseese.) That hockey plair, Alexander Sol Henderson, he jist up and defecated over to our side, like the old Stallion's dotter dun. I think if the hole Rossian team done that and sot asylums with yer Tronto Toreasses, we'da hadda good chants in that Roosia-Canda Serious.

Jip Ann: Cap: TUKYUH. Cheef Xport: Munny. Cheef Import: Us. These little fellas has compleated the Grand Uncle Slam by beatin' yer Yanks to the draw-strings on the publick's purrse. They've transvesterized alla us with ther raddios and give most of us a Toyola Cornary. And now they're comin' over here with ther Nixxon cameras and takin' pitchers of us quaint North Amerkan pessants in our natif costooms. They've alreddy started buyin' up yer French shattos, yer Callfornya wineros, and our Bertish Columbyan woods ... won't be long before they own all the forst fires we got.

Kareer: Still in subdivishuns, even after that wore where we all got brane-washed by Gennul M'Carthy. We went over ther to free our Seoul brothers, and now, by golly, they're in a worse repressed state than ever.

Chiner: Cap: PEEKIN. One of the reesins the wife and I jist had the one issyuh, Orville, is that sumbuddy told us that every second child born in the wirld today is Chinee, and we dint think the naybors wud unnerstand. Mind you, the child wudha grow'd up to be offal civillyized, fer yer Chinee was ritin' pomes on note-paper wen we was trynta rub Flintstones togither in a cave fer to be in heat. They had a wall-to-wall country when the rast of us was Neeandertall to a grasshopper.

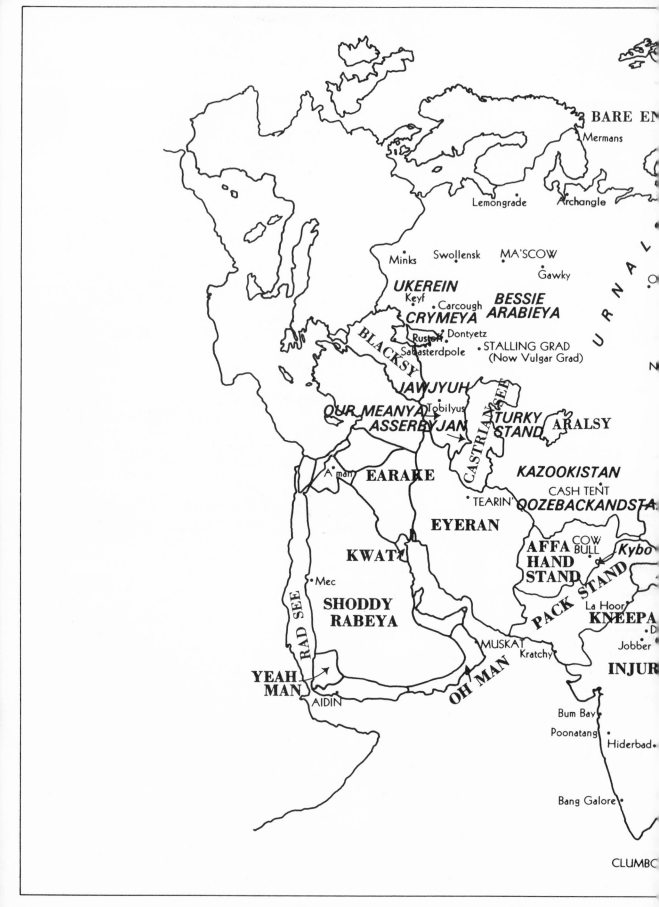

Yer Azure

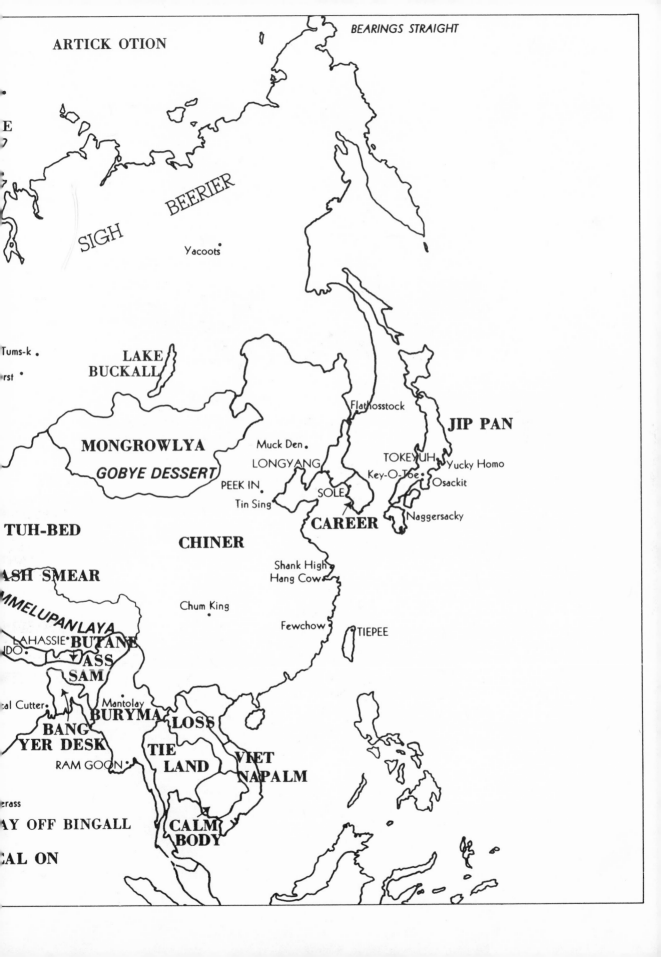

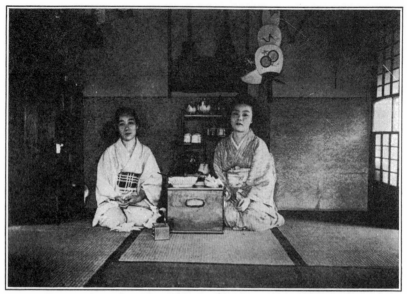

Geeseya girls

I dunno if you seen them Chinee Exhibishunists we had at yer Royl. (I don't meen your Winter's Fare. I meen yer Ontaryo Musuleum, wher they keeps yer Eejipjin Mummys and the Dinashores.) Well sir, they brung in a lode of Chiney horses was so fulla life-like it wudha made you think you was in the trots with Harvey Feely-on. And they had a prinsess in a jaded soot giftrapped with gold ribbons . . . I don't say it was comfurbull . . . musta give her an offal crack of a hernya . . . but my gol she was laid out in stile on her beer.

So if, as they say, yer wirld is to be took over by yer Yellow Perls, at leese we'll be koncord with hy-stile. Them fellas got a slant on life with more culcher in it than a Okey cheese what's old enuff to eet yer bred.

Tie-one: Cap: TYPE-A. This is John's other Chinamen. Not the ones run by Masty Tung and Joe N. Lye and them other nonnyginaryans. This iland is run by Shanky Shek, who'se even more jerry-attrick, and got famuss mostly by marryin' one of yer Soong sisters (I don't mind wich one . . . Maxine, Patty er Laverne).

Hung Kong: Cap: VICTEROLIA. Wher yer soots is maid wile you wait on yer stoppovers. The wife she had a chants to git a paira slax brung back fer her by a toorist cussin, but she was 'fraid the fly mite be sowed on sidewaze.

Veet Napalm: Another peece of trubble. After yer Yank pullout, yer Sygones wasn't 'sposed to be Hannoyed by yer gorillas in black pajamas. I gess our peacemakers shud git back there and rafferee. But I think they got pretty badly bugged wen they had to ware them shorts rite there in yer jungle's mouth.

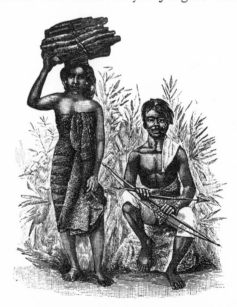

Girl and boy Maylay

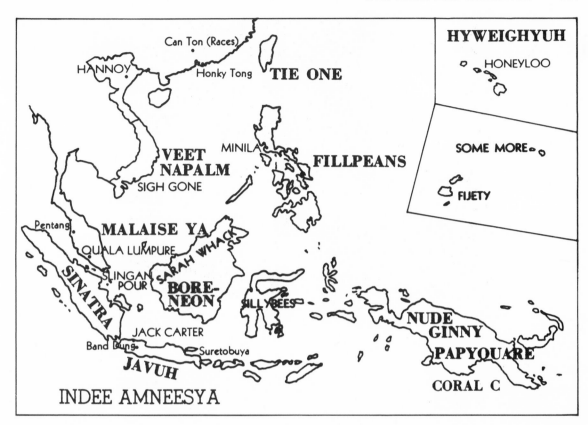

Southeest Azure

Louse: Is a manny splinterd thing.

Tieland: Not the store at Bloor and Yung, but the place where the King and I lived. (Cap: Bungcock.) Toorists who go ther love it. Gits thim rite between the tempels.

Cambodyuh: Cap: UNPERNOUNCIBLE. Wunder if they miss them Amerkans now that they don't git bommed every nite?

Malaisesya: Cap: COALA LUMPER. Is reely the old Brit. colony of Maylaya, pluss North Barnyo and Sarahwhacks. After a not-so-sibil war, they took ther Lumpers and formed up a fedreeation, even tho' sum of the parts is split by bawdys of water. They mines yer tins and smelts it, too. And they gotta lotta rubber plants.

Slinganpour: Cap: Ditto. Had the declairation of the interdependents in '65 after suffrin' with Malaiseya fer a cuppla yeers.

Indy-amnesia: Cap: JAK CARTER. All got together after yer war and Dutchclensed therselves. Was Bornyo yestiddy (the part that warn't Maylayed), Sinatra, Bally, yer Sillybees, and a Archpellycan of other eyelets . . . pluss some Java.

Fillpeans: Cap: QUEEZY-ON-SITTY. (Reely? I'll take Manilla.) Should be called yer Marshal Ilands, on accounta that's th'only way they can deel with yer Huckster, a vulcannic groop of Ilanders hoo kept things hot fer thim by continyally 'rupptin'.

Hwyuh: Cap: HONEYLOOLOO. State Flour: Hi-biscits. Is a buncha Corral Reefer Ilands, oney one of wich is called by that name. The rest has names like Mowee (!) and Wahoo (!), wich gives you sum idee wat goes on ther. They've bin bommed ever sints them Jap Kamistakazoo pile-its give 'em a sneek prevue of World War II . . . but then that's the Hwy-yin War Chants you take.

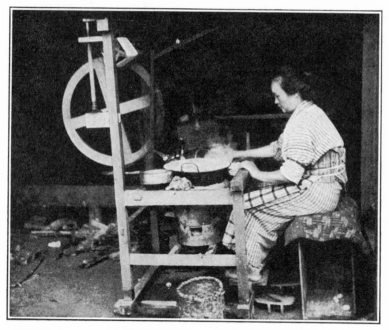

Noodle worker unwinding

They has sevril vullcanoes on yer active list, bein' not that fur Eest of Krackyertoa. Best noan of ther smokers is probly Moanin Low. Toorists wud be safer with yer Dime-a-hed, wich is the same thing, only ex-stink. But why not mingle with yer serfs on yer beech at Whykicky and git leid, wich is a luvly way of bean alohaded down by puttin' flours on you well before you passes on.

Bermer: Cap: RAMGOON. Talk about perspitation wetness, you ask anybuddy served in yer Windgate Champain agin yer Jap. Yer thunder comes up like Don on yer roda Mantolay durin' yer mudsoon seizin. And yer avrage bivvy-whacked footslogger offen found nothin' between hisself and the ground but a thin natif wooman.

Injer: Cap: NUDE ELLY. Run by Miz Gandy and her dansers, who wares the durbins round ther heds and the dypers round ther middles and kin charm the rattle offa Co-Bra. Jist reesently they bin havin' a blast at our expense and turnin' into atomical bums. And it was us in Canda that's bin helpin' them with ther Nukyuler piles. You'd think all them Seek peeple wud be too bizzy fightin' off fammin and berth control fer to take all that time out fer the Nukuler fishin.

They never seem to have enuff food at ther Noo Delly. I think we shudda bin shippin' them our surplices of markus

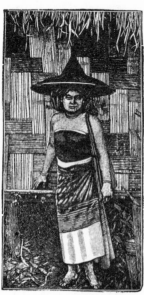

Hukstress

wheet, instedda bildin' up yer react-shunarys from yer Coballts. Ya'd think they'd druther have a full boll a rice rather'n a cuppla mega-tuns of mushroom clowd.

Seal-on: Cap: C'LUMBO. Has a lady Prime Mistress like Injuh. And an even better tee service without yer cast sistem, wich they got rid of. (It was tuk up by Hollo-wood, Callfornya, wher all the lemons comes from.)

Packstand: Cap: KRATCHY. This bunch'd be yer Muslins, yer Punjabbers, and yer Parslees. Langridge spoke is Ird-doo, and writ is yer Samscript. Mosta yer culcher come from yer Moe-gulls, who spent all ther time around LaHore. (The wife sez that may be fizzcal, but it's not culcher.)

Bangyerdesk: Cap: DECKER. Cheef Crop: Reckerd ranefall. Cheef Import: Fornade. The intire place is at the delter formed by yer Gangreen and yer Brama-putrid Rivers. The hole basen is poorly draned, 'speshully during yer monsoors, and the only ups in the place is yer Chittygangbang Hills.

Bhutane: Cap: TIM POO. Has the famuss Festerall of A Thousand Lites, after wich it is throne away. But, fer a buck .79, it's a pritty good festerall.

Siccim: Cap: GANGTALK. Where Injians go during the dog daze . . . and end the evenin' with a Bhang.

Nepple: Cap: CATMANDOO. The home of Mount Everset in yer Himmelupan-layas. Differnt tribes are yer Gerkins and yer Bra Men. Also yer Sherpys, incloodin' that Tent Sing who reeched his peek in '53 under Sir Edmound Hilly.

Tuh-bed: Cap: LeHASSLE. Home of yer Dolly Lamba, 'til yer Chinee c'lectivized yer monks into one big co-opulative. But yer T'betters don't worry, fer they bleeves in yer ree-incarseration. They figger they'll be back in yer lama-saddle agin retro-activly, long's they keep workin' ther Dile-a-Prare weels. As the most ellvated peeple in the wirld, ther used to livin' under lotsa pressyour.

Cashsmear: One of yer seven Vales that yer Packy and yer Injin has a hellabaloo, skindo, and Jammu sessyn over evry once in a wile.

Affagrandstand: Cap: COWBULL. Jist t'other side of Injure up yer Hindoo's Kush'n thru yer Kybo Pass. Cheef Ocku-pathan: Ridin' fast hoarses and speering the ring in eech other's nozes.

Ear-ran: Capital: UNLIMITED. Home of them Purrzyan cats who got well-fixed wen ther Shaw sunk his shaft and got well-oiled. Most famuss old-time Ear-runner is Omar yer Tensemaker, Rug-cutter, and Singer of Songs. D'you mind "Omar, he's makin' eyes at me" and "Jist a jug, and a thou, and you by my side loafin' in the wildness"?

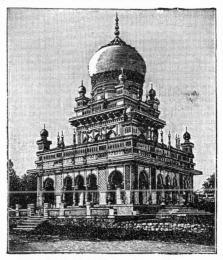

Taj Mahar (leev shoos outside)

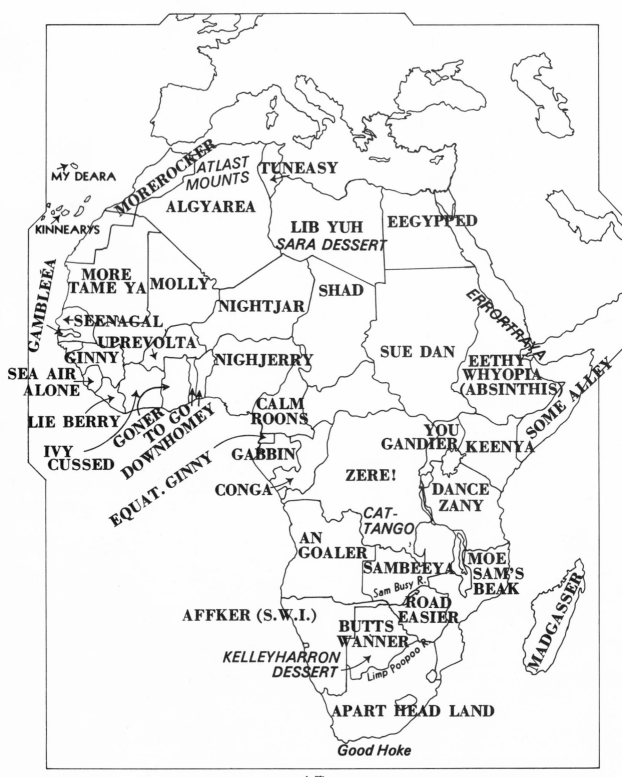

MY DEARA

KINNEARYS

MOREROCKER

ATLAST MOUNTS

TUNEASY

ALGYAREA

LIB YUH
SARA DESSERT

EEGYPPED

GAMBLEEA

MORE TAME YA

MOLLY

SHAD

NIGHTJAR

SEENAGAL

ERRORTRAYA

UPREVOLTA

GINNY

NIGHJERRY

SUE DAN

EETHY WHYOPIA (ABSINTHIS)

SEA AIR ALONE

LIE BERRY

CALM ROONS

IVY CUSSED

GONER TO GO DOWNHOMEY

EQUAT. GINNY

GABBIN

CONGA

YOU GANDIER

KEENYA

SOME ALLEY

ZERE!

DANCE ZANY

CAT-TANGO

AN GOALER

SAMBEEYA

MOE SAM'S BEAK

Sam Busy R.

AFFKER (S.W.I.)

ROAD EASIER

BUTTS WANNER

MADGASSER

KELLEYHARRON DESSERT

Limp Poopoo R.

APART HEAD LAND

Good Hoke

Affker

AFFKER

It's allus bin called yer Dark contnint, not so much doo to the culler of ther skins, but on accounta the dark deeds yer white man has dun there in yer used-peeple trade. It started as soon as C'lumbus had his Day in Amurka. Furst it was yer Injians was given yer slave bracelets. But they dint take to hard work and tuk to ther grave insted. So yer overseezers thot it wud be better if they got some imports fer to do it . . . and yer Affkans was chose as yer Noo Wirld's first dis-pleased persons. And if ya wonder why they're still feelin' that way in the big sitties today, jist mind the old saying: "As yer raped, so shall ye sow."

More-ocko: Cap: RABIT. Is bound to be 'memberd fer all them moovys that has brung in so much over yer Cashbar . . . "Castablanket" with Ingland Bergmar and Humpy Gocart, "Tanjeer," and "Marrowketch." Rabit has bin scene by most peeple in transit, and even yer Fez is familliar. Cheef Export: Havin' the re-runs on the TV.

Al-jeerya: Cap: ALCHEERS. Between them two names is the story of the last twenny yeers rite there. Yer natif was so tired of bein' Frenched he got revolting, so he was jumped on from a grate hite by yer Paristroopers. Grand Charlie the Gall thot 'bout freeing Cuebec, but he give up and, insted, freed yer Alcheerios with a reeferendum. They ben Bellacose ever sints, sept the wimmen, hoo still lives with a veil of tiers. Ther's no happy Bo-mediann fer them.

Twoneezya: Cap: TUNAS. Fulla old Roamin roons. I don't meen yer middle-ages Eyetallyans. I meen yer B.C. Roamin who left his Aqueducks all over the place durin' his Puny-ick wars agin yer Carta-Ginny-Hens.

Libby-ugh: Cap: BIN-GASSY. Another Arrid spot around yer Arb-pits. Trubble with Norse Affker, it's like a sosser that's bin blowed, but the wet stuff all fell on the rim and there's nuthin' left fer yer senter.

(The rim bein' yer Atlast Mounts, and the senter yer Sarah.) A lot of yer Wirld War II was fot here chasin' Genrl Ruml and his Aferka Corpses from yer hauls of old Montgummery to yer shores of Tripple-E.

Ther's still alotta fite left in Libyah. Ther leeder, Kernel Godaffy, was so ank-shuss to fite Isreeal, he coodn't wait and had a altered-caisson with yer Eejupshuns first.

Eegypped: Cap: KYRO. Did ya see on the TV the deception that Pressdent-that-was Nixxon got when he druv down yer Kyro main stem with Amoor Sedate? I think now that Tricksy's resined hisself, he'll more'n likely come back here and run fer Sfinks.

Suedan: Cap: CARTOMB. You look up yer Sores of yer Nile, and you'll be in the backseet of yer Suedan. Prinspal produck is gum Arbic, wich is wat the lokals do wen ther not chewin' the fat er fasin' Decca at 5 o'clock.

They're an indypendant bunch. They got thers from Egipped in '56, and by '70 they fot with therselves so hard they purt neer split agin. Sounds like us Irish on Sardy nites.

Etherwhyopenya: Cap: HADUSABAB-BY. Used to be called Abyssinya in all th'old familyer places. B'longd to yer Queen of Sheeper, but now to a Empurer hoo calls hisself yer Lyin of Judo and hoo has, up till now, bin thot to be Hylee Satissfackery. But it looks like he'll be taken fer a constitootional.

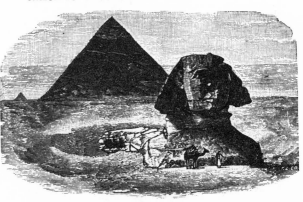

Peer amid finks

Some-alley: Cap: MUGGERDISCO. The place where a cuppla our flyers was captivated after they'd bin roled in Some-Alley and seen ther Errortraya.

Shad: Cap: FORT LARMEE. (Sounds Y-oming, don't it?) You've herd the expressyun "brown as a Shad's belly"? Well sir, this Shad itself she varrys from hot and tord to hot and horid. It ain't the heat, it's the humanity. And I dunno how they stan' it.

Up Revolta: Cap: OOGADOOGOO. Sound like baby talk, and mebbe that's cuz few of them will git a chants to grow up. They got a drout on now makes Saskatchewin in yer 30s seem like yer Garden of Eatons.

Nightjar: Ditto.

Molly: Is fulla berbers, wich is why its tale is cut short.

Moreattainya: All washed up. Used to be a ship.

Seenagal: Everybuddy works fer peenuts . . . and that's exackly what they gits.

Ginny: Sounds like a Eyetalian colny, but it were French. They was the ones come to danse in Tronto with no brassears, and the hole thing was a big bust.

See-air Lee-own: Cap: FREE TOWN. Was called yer white man's grave, but things is improved. Now all men is cremated equal.

Lie Beerier: Cap: MANOVERYUH. After Linken freed yer slaves, they wanted ther own Continental back. By 1930, they was enslaverin' eech other agin. Jist reesently, the Ewe Ass promised to assist them fiscally. Let's hope Ford don't turn out to be a Edsell.

Ivy Coast: Sounds like ther in leeg with Yail and Harvered, but brite stoogents here get to go to yer Sorebone (in Paris, Fran's).

Goner: Wen it was Birtish, it wur called yer Gold Coste. But them Anglish bullyonairs musta took it all with 'em. Cap: Acrid.

Downhomey: They got a rotatin' Prime Minster. Everybuddy's got problems. We're still tryna get our Primester to keep both feet on the ground.

Nigerearia: Pritty well recuvvered from being Bi'affered in 1970. Yer two fackshuns used a daring new techneek . . . furgiveness.

Camroons: Sounds Scots, but is micksed French and Anglish like us. They git along fine, and they're all the one culler jist like us, only differnt.

Gaboon: Not the munky with the red and blue buttum, but the place neer wher Al Switzer, the organist hoo woodn't hurt a fly, set up his hosspittle at Langrene.

Conga: Cap: BRAZZIERVILL. This ain't yer old Bulgin Conga, but a small ex-Frenched obsessyun.

Zere! Cap: KINSHAFTYA, farmerly Layaboldville. Yer Bulgin-Conga-that-was. This is the place where everybuddy got Ubangeed about, includin' yer mishnarys . . . and even yer mercymarys. Reesin they had all the trubble in the last place was it were discuvvered in the first place by that grate exploiter, Layapalled First, yer Bulgin King, noan to his intmit fiends as Leo-in-the-Sky-with-Dymonds. A pure xample of sowing wat you have raped.

Ugandier: Cap: KOMPELLA. Jist th' oppsit from a royl white man bein' opprussive. Here, it's a natif sarjint who gits permoted by the Bertish into an offser's mess and ends up as the lokal genral God . . . Amen.

Keenyuh: Cap: NOROBEY. They're a quiet, flyswattin' bunch now. But do you mind wen they was revoltin' under the Sophy of Tucker, the last of the redhot Maumaus?

Tannedzany: Cap: DERE IS ALAM. Grate seenery on yer grate Lakes . . . Victoriuss, Tanglenecker, and Myassa. Hi point is Mount Killamansorrow, but don't miss yer Serene-getto Nashnul Park, where all the animals is preserved as games and you can still see rhinosasserases and hippy-optimists. But stay in yer car, or they'll come where you are.

Zammbeya: Cap: LOOSEACTERS. Like Genral Allmeen of Ugandy, Pressdent Ken Kowunder give his Injians reservations on the next plane. They also dis-

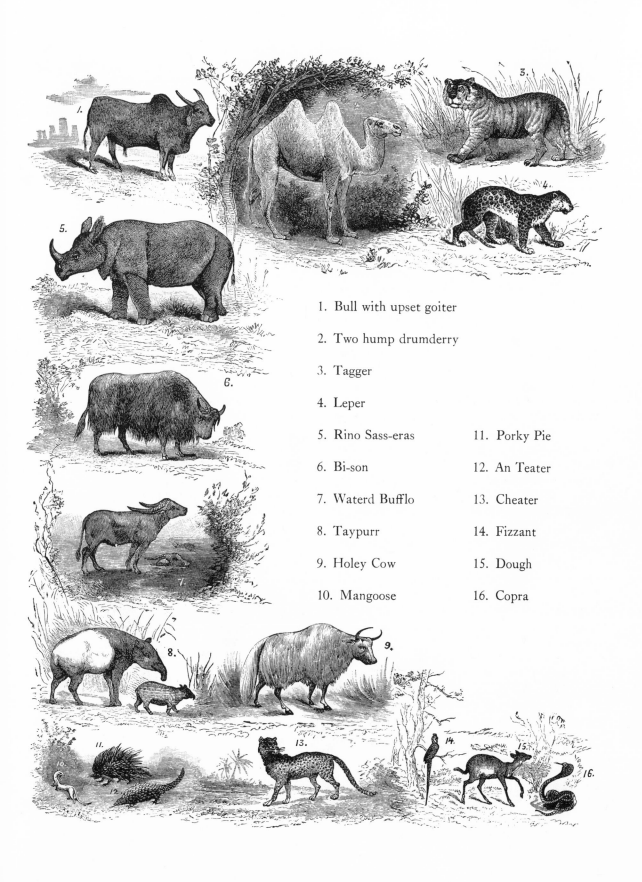

1. Bull with upset goiter

2. Two hump drumderry

3. Tagger

4. Leper

5. Rino Sass-eras

6. Bi-son

7. Waterd Bufflo

8. Taypurr

9. Holey Cow

10. Mangoose

11. Porky Pie

12. An Teater

13. Cheater

14. Fizzant

15. Dough

16. Copra

courge Canajian toorism in the worst way, but so far our Depart of Eternal Affairs hasn't lifted a V-toe agin them.

Moe Sam Beak: Sounds like yer Three Scrooges, but it's one of yer Porchgeese that's reddy to jump offa the Porch and stop bein' sich a geese.

Mallowme: Lies on the edge of yer Rift Valley . . . like alla us marred men in yer silent majororyty!

Angoaler: Cap: LOU-UNDER. Used ta be Porchgeese Wist Affker. Was uncoverd in 1482, and yer Lispin murchant went rite into yer slave trade fer the next cupple hundert yeers. ("Our product is stealin', our strenth is peeple.") Wen the place got depopillated by this kinda export trade, yer Porchgeese moved in fur coffee, wich they wud take after yer first native up-risin' in the mornin'. Jist reesently, yer Porchgeese hadda change of guvmint and a change of hart, so we expect Angle-Lola will soon be goin' thru the changes fer the bettors.

Roadeasier: Cap: SOL'SBERRY. Mane inderstree seams to be splittin'. They split off from yer North Roadeeziers (now yer Zambeans) in '64, but staid in yer Come-on-Welth. Then Britten sujjested they give ther black peeple a little more of yer universal sufferage. (My gol, haven't them pore peeple had enuff . . . do they have to go thru more suffrageyet?) So Eon Smith 'n his tropickal whites broke from offa our fambly of nayshuns, and in

retalian-eye-ation us Bertish Umpirers dropped ther Fornade and set up yer Blockaid. Yer Untiedyed Nations wanted Number 10 Downer Street to throw them over by force, but Ted Heath was too bizzy toorin' with his band.

Funny thing, yer white Supreems under Eon and the rast of the Smith brothers is nowdaze considerd modrits. And they is, too, compaired to yer white Souse Affkans acrost yer Limp-poopoo River.

Soused Affker: Cap: PREE-TORY. TV er not TV—that used to be the quastion. Sept in yer Southest of yer Affkers, wher it's jist now comin' in with yer Dick Van's dyke and yer Looseheel Balls.

You take yer boobs on the toobs, the wife she'll sit up all Friedy nites watching them late late moovys on yer Chanel Number 3 . . . "The Thing that Ate Boston," "Tarzin and yer Water-bugs," and "Drackoolah Drinks the Bride of Frank'n Steen." Meself, I can't be botherd with all that bubble-gum fer the eyes. But wen it cums to yer noos, I likes to see fer myself jist how bad the wirld reely looks. It was yer Veet Napalm war bein' on the TV every nite that finely led to its bein' stopped, not becuz of yer politickals promesses.

So wut's this got to do with yer peeple of Caketown and Joe's Hamberg, and yer Bandtoostand Townships? Jist that a nayshun that's bin afraid to have the TV is afraid to hold a mira up to therselves.* And that to me, is yer Sousaffker Story. Aparthed is sich sweet sorrow?

*RESINED FEETNOTE: And I don't blame them bean afraid of "Let's Make a Deal," cuz that's how yer hole U.S. Presdenshul sistem seems to have bin run the last few yeers.

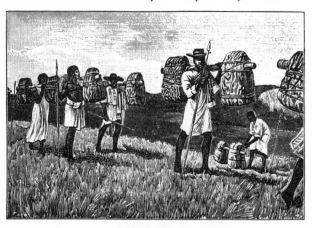

Aferkins afairy

TAKIN' STOCK: YER CONCLUSSIONS

I sed at the beginnin' that Jogfree was wat we had to start with, and Histry is the mess we all maid of it. So now we bin all around the wirld, wat are we gonta do 'bout the mess?

YER GLOWBALL POINTA VUE

Ther's two kindsa peeple in yer whirld: passmists and optometrists. The first sez we're all hedded fer Hell in a han-kar, and the secunt sez eet, drink, and be, Mary, for tomorra ther'll be a guvmint surplice. Yer Pessymissed was lately orgy-nized into yer Clubbed of Rome, and it insests that as the day goes by to yer yeer 2000 (yer start of yer next millenema), we'll all be livin' in a Doomed Stadyum. Yer Optummyists say that kinda tock has bin around for decayeds. Accorn to a 1944 report, we was s'posed to have run outa tin, nickels, led, zink, and mangyneeze by 1974. Dint happen by a long shot, and we got more copper than we kin shake a nitestick at. Pert neer 200 yeer ago, Tomass Malthused sed we'd run outa fud if we dint keep killin' each other off with wore, fammin, 'n pustulence. And yer pessaryists wud say that's sackly wat we bin doin'. But most of our decreases in yer popillation has bin from pullin' out to avoid the issyou.

Yer Berth Controll: Peeple gittin' togither with peeple fer begettin' other peeple is one of yer sore-spots of underrest. We was oney 2 billyuns in 1945, but come next yeer weel be about dubbled up. Mebbe we'll have to teech yer undeeveloped nayshuns with ther over-deeveloped famlees how to cupple without dubblin' up. Wurds won't do it . . . we may have to draw them a diafram.

Mind you, you take yer Pope Pall, he din't help much wen he woodn't let his rithim band have the Emasculate Contraseption. Bein' Inflailabull is nice fer him, but I don't think everybuddy cud foller that method. Yer vasextummists garntee a stitch in time saves nine munth. But the wife and I is too odd fashunned fer that. Fer instinks, we has never voted Libral since they aloud yer homeysexuals to have the free abortions.

Yer Chants Ya Takes: Peeple is not th'only wild cards in our deck. You ask any Prime-mary Pro-juicer wether his bizness deep-ends on the wether, and he'll show you his polissy fer Crap Insurients. This spring is a good xample. We had forty daze of rain, follered by yer 'lection (sixty daze of hot air). And I dunno wich was wurst, but it sure brung out yer grassed-hopper, yer catterdeepiller, yer Japnee Beatle,* and yer Army wurm from Camp Boredom.

Now you sitty folkers may not be too consarned about a few slugs wen yer sittin' by yer swimpool on yer Assteroterf. But you mite be bugged by all this later on when you has to pay mebbe sixty sents fer yer loafa yer crack er yer hole weet bred.

Yer Short-edges: Too much munny chasin' too few goodies . . . sounds like sailers on leeve, but it's reely our plite to-day. Sum of yer short-edges is nacheral. There's not too much Western lam around on accounta yer Coy-oatees has been lickin' our chops before we gits them to slotter. Now there's some is tryna pass a law to pertect Ky-otes as a indanger speeces. But I think it's best to seprate yer sheap from yer wolf, becuz if they lay down together, it's yer wolf that gits up again. I think yer avrage Ecky-ollygist tries to

*CONDUCKTED FEETNOTE: I don't mean that Sez-you Oshawa used to wave his stick at yer Trontuh Sympathy Orchester.

pass a law nowadaze every time a loon gits a mygrain from a out-bored mutter.

Yer Derry End: Sumtimes yer problem is not natcheral, but jist man doin' it to man. Cupple yeers ago, our aig prices dropt so bad (29 sents the duz) that it wernt even wurthwile cleenin' them off. So yer. Common House thot they'd raze prices by lowerin' aig perduckshun. Well wat they dun was like cuttin' off yer nose to spike yer drink, fer they slottered hens holesail . . . and not fer the pot, jist fer the plot. Berried them in thousands . . . they was all gassed at the time. (I mean yer hen, not nessairly yer Em Pees.)

That's how our guvmint used to deel with yer Ovary-produckshun. But not that Aggravaculcher Minster we got now, Youjean Whalebone. A lotta peeple think he perteckts us farmers too much, but my gol, that's his job, that's what he was give the post fer . . . to scratch our backs.

I had my own aig problems this spring. Bein' 'lection time, we had a lotta wind, and in March it was purt near a hoory-cane. (Blew mother's hat agin the barn and held her ther fer a week.) One of our hens stood with her back to that wind and laid the same aig six times. You'll never make munny that way, 'less you cut down yer overhed.

And you take yer milk supports. (I don't meen them things the Wimmen's Libbriums burned wen they started ther movemint. I meen the guvmint help that hasn't so far seemed to cleer the derry air.) And with them Krafty peeple about, it's not even wirthwile fer to cut the cheese. Every day more'n more fine up-standin' Holsteen farmers gits outa the derry bizness cuz ther tired of gittin' up at five o'clock seven day a week, grabbin' a holt of a hunnert and twenny tits, and gittin' them hosed and stripped.

You mark my book, there's gonna be a ring-taled snorter of a milk short-edge. That's why all these restrunts is gittin' topfull watetrusses. Peeple is tired of them inedible oils in ther cawfee and wants the reel thing. Most sitty peeples was bottle babys from the start and niver did git to know the plessures of draft. Or corpulent punnishmint neether. And that's why today the new degeneration is roamin' up and down Yung Street lookin' fer a Mass-use parler that rubs you the rong way. You don't see any farm boys hangin' around them places lookin' fer a slap on the back-forty or a bust in the mouth . . . they've had it all, long before ther puberty pogram . . . and with a barn fulla nood animals to boot.

But I'm thinkin' of givin' up cows and keepin' bees insted. It's less spase, and you don't have to cleen out yer hives twice a day. Besides, I've bin stung every other way ther is.

Yer Beef: I s'pose the biggest beef is still yer Beef. You probly wonder wat's rong with forced-feedin' wen you bin doin' it to yer kids every mornin' at breckfist? Mind you, yer not shovin' in the horemoans, like yer DES, wich Duz everything to mice, includin' the canser.

Yer Biggar Beef: If you took the trubble to Gallup anybuddy's Pole, I gess the Number One consarn wud be yer Inflay-shun. It jist seems to keep creepin' up on us like that symphetic Nylin undyware. Did ya know that on accounta yer Laws of Supplize and Demanned that we has dubbled our amounta munny sints 1964?

Now the only safe way to dubble munny is to fold it once and put it back in yer pocket. But guvmints all over has bin printin' the stuff like they was contra-fitters. It's to pay fer all that defecat spendin' they do. (Yer defecat is wat you've got wen youse haven't got as much as if youse jist had nothin'.) Ya see, yer guvmint don't have to keep book . . . they jist throw it at the voaters every four yeer. That's why evry guvmint estimat contanes a extry estimit of how much more it's gonna cost than yer ridge-in-all estimit. This allows yer guvmint to go round fiskaly unbalanced. If you er I tryed that, we'd end up in jail bank-rupchered.

Yer Catch: The reel trubble is nobuddy

likes inflammation exsept guvmints. They kin pay off ther detts cheeper, becuz the munny they borried in the first place is wirth so much less now. So they keeps on borryin' more, instedda the unpoplar way of razin' munny—taxass. Mane problem rite now in Canda is that yer provinshuls and yer Feds havn't figgerd out yet how to carve us all up fer revnoose . . . cant deeside on who duz wat with witch and to hoom.

Yer politickles is afrayed that if we stopped inflayshun rite now, our posterity wud disappeer, and we'd be back in our deep Depressyun. But mosta us pore devels wooden notiss sich a thing, becuz deprest is the way we've alweez lived. It's yer pore and yer old that's reely bin fixed by all that out-go on ther in-cums. And if sumbuddy was to say "Let 'em eet cake," well it's purty much the same price as yer loafer bred. And I think by this time next yeer yer bred and cakes will both have gone the way of all flesh. All the meat we'll eet will be a can of Doctor Ballhards.

So wat's to be dun about it? Shood we save er spend? If you gane on the swingers, do you loose on the rustabouts? Seems to me, eether way is like bangin' yer stones aginst a wall. I think we're on the horns of a pairaducks. Bast thing to do probly is buy a ticket on the Olimpric Lottery got up by yer Mare Jeans Drop-out. I know it's a chants fer a millyun, but I garntee it's honist, fer the hole rang-dang-doo is run by yer compewter. And I say you kin allus trussed a cumpeweter, becuz it's sumbuddy that, tho' he works in the sitty, he lives with us in the country.

Other'n that, I'm 'frayed the plane trooth is that we have to grab yer bulls by the tale, pull in our horns, and back off a bit. That meens we have to lern to want less, not moar. Becuz the next inncreases in yer hy cost of keepin'-up-livin' may be the straws up the camel that broke the banks. We jist have to stop bein' so Gross about our Nashnull Produck.

*   *   *

Ther's just wan oinkmint on yer fly I shud menshun. And that's the possbility of yer nookieleer holycost.

Up 'til reecent, mosta us thot the danger of fall-off had faln off. But the whirld is so neuralgic fer th'old days of the Fiftys that all the golden oldys are bein' brot back. Fer eggsample, twenny year ago yer Tronto Transports went outa Cmission, and yer teeny-age Exhibitionist wuz swimmin' the Lake. We bin so brane-washed by them good ole daze, I wooden be s'prised if they brung back yer Kareen war.

And now, mebby, it's Hero-shimmy time agen. That's why everybuddy wants to git into yer tomic reeacter bizness. And Canda seams to be yer mane supplyer . . . we bin doon deels with Injure, Archintinny, Soused Kareer, and the Lord nose hoo-all sub yer rosy.

If the only way we got to beet yer inflayshun and yer over-popillation is by turnin' the hole wirld into a pile a atomical bums, then this is in deed . . .

. . . YER END.

INDECKS

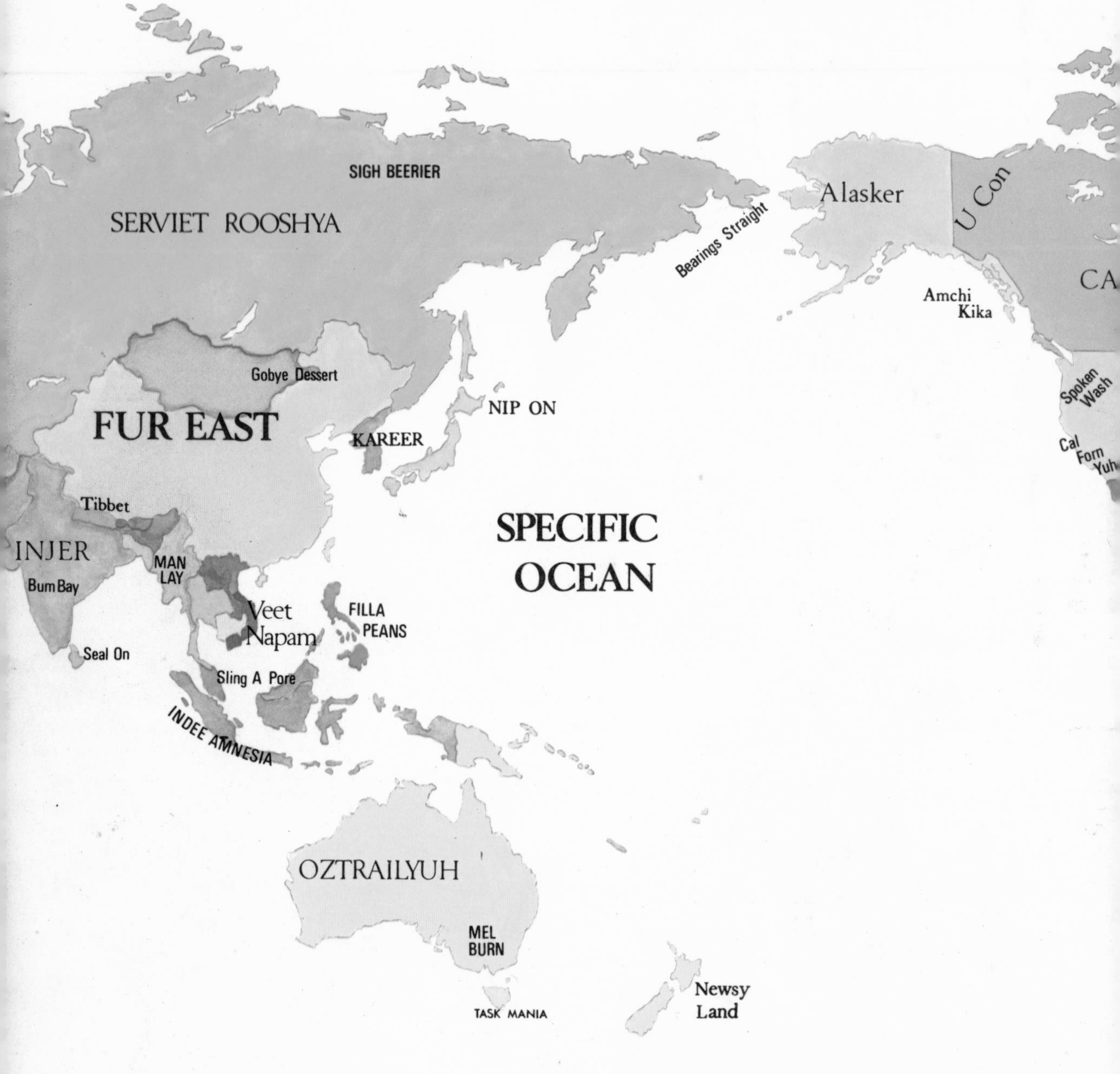

SIGH BEERIER

SERVIET ROOSHYA

Alasker

U Con

Bearings Straight

CA

Amchi
Kika

Gobye Dessert

FUR EAST

Spoken
Wash

NIP ON

KAREER

Cal
Forn
Yuh

Tibbet

**SPECIFIC
OCEAN**

INJER

MAN
LAY

Bum Bay

Veet
Napam

FILLA
PEANS

Seal On

Sling A Pore

INDEE AMNESIA

OZTRAILYUH

MEL
BURN

Newsy
Land

TASK MANIA